ENDOCRINOLOGY RESEARCH AND CLINICAL DEVELOPMENTS

T0293169

IMPAIRED GLUCOSE TOLERANCE AND INSULIN RESISTANCE

RISK FACTORS, MANAGEMENT AND HEALTH IMPLICATIONS

ENDOCRINOLOGY RESEARCH AND CLINICAL DEVELOPMENTS

Additional books in this series can be found on Nova's website
under the Series tab.

Additional e-books in this series can be found on Nova's website
under the e-book tab.

ENDOCRINOLOGY RESEARCH AND CLINICAL DEVELOPMENTS

IMPAIRED GLUCOSE TOLERANCE AND INSULIN RESISTANCE

RISK FACTORS, MANAGEMENT AND HEALTH IMPLICATIONS

SANDRA WAGNER
EDITOR

New York

Copyright © 2015 by Nova Science Publishers, Inc.

Library of Congress Cataloging-in-Publication Data

ISBN: 978-1-63483-085-0
Library of Congress Control Number: 2015941527

Published by Nova Science Publishers, Inc. † New York

Contents

Preface

The prevalence of type 2 diabetes mellitus (T2DM) has been increasing worldwide, and it is becoming a public health concern. In this book, the pathophysiological risk factors of progression from normoglycemia to prediabetes and the lifestyle modifications and pharmacological interventions for preventing or delaying the development of glucose intolerance is examined. Furthermore, the insulin signaling pathway regulates the cellular uptake of glucose and wholebody metabolic homeostasis in mammalians. This book explores the improvement of estrogen signaling in preventing the comorbidities of insulin resistance. The next chapter focuses on nutritional management during the perioperative period, focusing on glucose metabolism and insulin sensitivity. There are three major problems for nutritional management during the perioperative period. These problems are addressed and suggestions are made on how to alleviate them. Finally, Cystic Fibrosis (CF) is the most common lethal inherited disorder in Caucasians, affecting 1 in 2,500 - 2,800 live births. The last chapter examines impaired glucose tolerance in cystic fibrosis.

Chapter 1 – The prevalence of type 2 diabetes mellitus (T2DM) has been increasing worldwide, and it is becoming a public health problem. Prediabetes is defined as a condition in which people have higher than normal blood glucose levels but not high enough to be diagnosed as T2DM. However, every year, approximately 5%–10% of people with prediabetes eventually develop T2DM. Lifestyle modification, a combination of diet and exercise, is an effective means of preventing the development of T2DM. Impaired fasting glucose (IFG), impaired glucose tolerance (IGT), and a combination of both are prediabetic states; each state represents different populations with overlapping subclinical characteristics and pathophysiological etiologies.

Patients with any of these prediabetic states have moderate to severe insulin resistance and impaired insulin secretion. IFG is characterized by severe hepatic insulin resistance with normal or near-normal muscle insulin resistance, whereas IGT is characterized by a marked muscle insulin resistance with only mild hepatic insulin resistance. Both conditions are characterized by a reduction in early-phase insulin secretion, while patients with IGT also have impaired late-phase insulin secretion. Recent studies on normoglycemic subjects indicate that elevated blood pressure and increased triglyceride or uric acid levels, resulting from weight gain, could be causes of reduction in insulin secretion and increase in insulin resistance. Therefore, weight loss, achieved with lifestyle modification, is important to improve insulin sensitivity and to preserve insulin-secreting capacity in order to prevent conversion from normoglycemia to prediabetes.

Similar to patients with T2DM, prediabetic patients have an increased risk of cardiovascular disease. Therefore, identification and intervention for individuals who are at high risk of prediabetes is a crucial first step in preventing a modifiable disease, and to save lives. This review aims to summarize the pathophysiological risk factors of progression from normoglycemia to prediabetes and the lifestyle modifications and pharmacological interventions for preventing or delaying the development of glucose intolerance.

Chapter 2 – The insulin signaling pathway regulates the cellular uptake of glucose and whole-body metabolic homeostasis in mammalians. Dysregulation of insulin secretion or alterations in the transduction of insulin receptor signal are associated with self-generating, progressive insulin resistance, which predisposes patients to a variety of life threatening chronic diseases. Activation of estrogen receptor (ER) signals by estrogen has beneficial effects on glucose homeostasis and energy metabolism by several pathways. Nevertheless, certain scientific results support that an overexpression of ER isoforms or hyperestrogenism may have important implications for the development of dysmetabolism, such as metabolic syndrome, type 2 diabetes and their comorbidities. Moreover, increased estrogen synthesis is erroneously supposed to disrupt the glucose uptake in the adipose tissue mass in obese patients and is presumed to contribute to insulin resistance and the associated comorbidities. By contrast, in animal experiments, pregnancy analogue estradiol administration improves the metabolic functions and exhibits cancer preventive capacity even in insulin resistant and obese ones. In human practice, multiparity associated good estrogen signaling shows strong tumor protective effect even against the cancers of highly hormone dependent female organs including overall breast cancer, endometrial and ovarian tumors. Considering the advantageous effects of suitable estrogen signaling on insulin secretion, cellular glucose uptake and further metabolic processes, estrogen administration seems to be a new therapeutic possibility to improve insulin sensitivity in patients with metabolic syndrome and diabetes mellitus.

Chapter 3 – Surgery is invasive, and injures the patient's physiology. Insulin resistance after surgery increases as the surgical procedure become extensive. Noxious stimuli activate sympathetic nerve system, causing inflammation. It also decreases the insulin sensitivity. Furthermore, hemodynamic changes caused by anesthesia, by bleeding from surgical procedure, and/or by hypothermia result in a stress.

After surgery, wound repair is required and the increase in catabolism must be kept minimal. In this view of point, appropriate nutritional management during perioperative period helps prevent catabolism. Blood glucose concentration was recognized recently as an important factor influencing to the outcome. Intensive insulin therapy, however, is not agreed is not upon universally. Shortage of glucose induces glyconeogenesis from amino acids and /or lipids, further causing extensive catabolism. For reducing this, glucose administration is important as well as a good static blood glucose level.

Protocols like ERAS (Enhanced Recovery After Surgery) were being proposed for quick recovery after surgery. This recommends drinking 400 mL of clear water containing carbohydrate 2 hours before anesthesia, but it does not include glucose administration during surgery. For prolonged surgery, patients obviously need good nutritional support. A small dose of glucose during surgery effectively suppresses ketogenesis, and attenuates postoperative insulin resistance.

In this chapter, the authors intend to describe the amount of carbohydrate required for the day of surgery, and the way to give carbohydrate. They propose a method of evaluating insulin sensitivity after surgery.

Chapter 4 – One of the major complications of Cystic Fibrosis (CF) is CF-related diabetes (CFRD) which increases in incidence with age, from 1-2% below the age of 10 years, to 25% in early adult life and over 50% in those above the age of 40 years.

The diagnosis of CFRD is made clinically or through the Oral Glucose Tolerance Test (OGTT) which measures elevation of the fasting or 2 hour blood glucose levels. The diagnosis of Impaired Glucose Tolerance (IGT) is made in those subjects with values between the normal and diabetic ranges. Outside of these definitions, abnormalities of the one hour glucose value of the

OGTT may also be present. In this review, the significance of IGT in the management of CF will be reviewed and areas requiring further research to manage IGT in CF will be highlighted.

In: Impaired Glucose Tolerance ...   ISBN: 978-1-63483-085-0
Editor: Sandra Wagner   © 2015 Nova Science Publishers, Inc.

Chapter 1

The Epidemiology and Management of Prediabetes: A Preventable Disease

Masanori Shimodaira, MD, PhD[*]

Department of Internal Medicine, Iida Municipal Hospital, Nagano, Japan

Abstract

The prevalence of type 2 diabetes mellitus (T2DM) has been increasing worldwide, and it is becoming a public health problem. Prediabetes is defined as a condition in which people have higher than normal blood glucose levels but not high enough to be diagnosed as T2DM. However, every year, approximately 5%–10% of people with prediabetes eventually develop T2DM. Lifestyle modification, a combination of diet and exercise, is an effective means of preventing the development of T2DM. Impaired fasting glucose (IFG), impaired glucose tolerance (IGT), and a combination of both are prediabetic states; each state represents different populations with overlapping subclinical characteristics and pathophysiological etiologies. Patients with any of these prediabetic states have moderate to severe insulin resistance and impaired insulin secretion. IFG is characterized by severe hepatic insulin

[*] Corresponding author: Masanori Shimodaira, MD, PhD. Address: 438 Yawata-machi, Iida, Nagano, 395-8502, Japan. Tel: +81 265-21-1255 (Ext. 7085), fax: +81 265-21-1266, e-mail: masanori19810813@yahoo.co.jp.

resistance with normal or near-normal muscle insulin resistance, whereas IGT is characterized by a marked muscle insulin resistance with only mild hepatic insulin resistance. Both conditions are characterized by a reduction in early-phase insulin secretion, while patients with IGT also have impaired late-phase insulin secretion. Recent studies on normoglycemic subjects indicate that elevated blood pressure and increased triglyceride or uric acid levels, resulting from weight gain, could be causes of reduction in insulin secretion and increase in insulin resistance. Therefore, weight loss, achieved with lifestyle modification, is important to improve insulin sensitivity and to preserve insulin-secreting capacity in order to prevent conversion from normoglycemia to prediabetes.

Similar to patients with T2DM, prediabetic patients have an increased risk of cardiovascular disease. Therefore, identification and intervention for individuals who are at high risk of prediabetes is a crucial first step in preventing a modifiable disease, and to save lives. This review aims to summarize the pathophysiological risk factors of progression from normoglycemia to prediabetes and the lifestyle modifications and pharmacological interventions for preventing or delaying the development of glucose intolerance.

Introduction

In the past few decades, the global incidence and prevalence of type 2 diabetes mellitus (T2DM) has dramatically increased in developed and developing countries alike. The total number of people with T2DM is projected to rise from 94 million in 2003 to 333 million in 2025 [1]. Given the increasing prevalence of T2DM and the high economic cost of treating the condition and its comorbidities, it is important to find effective ways of targeting individuals who are most at risk of developing the disease [2].

Prediabetes is defined as a state of abnormal glucose homeostasis characterized by impaired fasting glucose (IFG), impaired glucose tolerance (IGT), and a combination of both (IFG and IGT). Prediabetes is considered the 'gray area' between normal glucose levels and diabetic levels. The transition from the early metabolic abnormality that precedes T2DM to overt T2DM may take many years. However, current estimates indicate that most individuals (approximately up to 70%) with such prediabetic states eventually develop T2DM [3-6]. Therefore, it is appropriate that the individuals who are at risk are identified and appropriately managed, to prevent the development of T2DM. However, prediabetes has no specific signs or symptoms and several studies have suggested long-term damage to end-organs associated with T2DM may start in prediabetes.

The aim of this review is to provide recent evidence of prediabetes, and to summarize the risk factors and the interventions for prevention of prediabetes.

1. Definition of Prediabetes

In healthy individuals, glucose homeostasis is tightly controlled, and the fasting plasma glucose (FPG) concentration is maintained within a very narrow range (70–90 mg/dL) [7]. The terms IGT and IFG refer to a metabolic stage intermediate between normal glucose homeostasis and diabetes, referred to as prediabetes. Diagnostic criteria for prediabetes have changed over the time and currently vary depending on the institution (Table 1).

In 1979, the National Diabetes Data Group (NDDG) defined IGT as FPG < 140 mg/dL and 2-h plasma glucose (2h-PG) values of 75 g-oral glucose tolerance test (OGTT) ranging from 140–199 mg/dL [8]. The term IFG was introduced in 1997, whereby FPG values from 110–125 mg/dL additionally differentiated the metabolic state between normal and diabetes [9]. World Health Organization (WHO) defined IGT as FPG < 126mg/dL and 2h-PG from 140–199 mg/dL, and IFG as FPG of 110–125 mg/dL (in the absence of IGT) [10]. In 2003, the American Diabetes Association (ADA) lowered the FPG threshold for IFG from 110 to 100 mg/dL, which optimized the sensitivity and specificity in predicting T2DM [11]. However, WHO did not change its previous recommendations, placing greater emphasis on 2h-PG values. Therefore, the definition of IGT is the same for ADA and WHO; IFG is defined as FPG of 100–125 mg/dL according to the ADA definition, whereas 110–125 mg/dL according to the WHO definition.

Glycated hemoglobulin (HbA1c) levels below 6.0% are associated with an increased risk for T2DM [12]. In 2010, ADA suggested that HbA1c levels between 5.7%–6.4% can also be used for the diagnosis of prediabetes [13]. However, the Canadian Diabetes Association has based its definition on a higher risk level and suggests a HbA1c level between 6.0%–6.4% as a diagnostic criterion for prediabetes [14].

HbA1c can be measured at any time of day and is more convenient than FPG or 2h-PG in a 75 g-OGTT. Moreover, HbA1c testing also avoids the problem of day-to-day variability of glucose values as it reflects the average plasma glucose concentration over the period of 2–3 months [15].

Therefore, these changes in using HbA1c for diagnosis are expected to facilitate identification of individuals at risk for T2DM who could benefit from intervention.

Table 1. Diagnostic criteria for prediabetes

Authority, year	plasma glucose and HbA1c levels
NDDG 1979	IGT
	FPG: < 140 mg/dL and 2h-PG: 140-199 mg/dL
ADA 1997	IGT
	FPG: < 140 mg/dL and 2h-PG: 140-199 mg/dL
	IFG
	FPG :110-125 mg/dL
WHO 1999 and 2006 (most recent)	IGT
	FPG: < 140 mg/dL and 2h-PG: 140-199 mg/dL
	IFG
	FPG :110-125 mg/dL and 2h-PG < 200mg/dL (if measured)
ADA 2003	IGT
	FPG: < 140 mg/dL and 2h-PG: 140-199 mg/dL
	IFG
	FPG :100-125 mg/dL
ADA 2010 (most recent)	IGT
	FPG: < 140 mg/dL and 2h-PG: 140-199 mg/dL
	IFG
	FPG :100-125 mg/dL
	HbA1c
	5.7 – 6.4% (a new category of high risk for diabetes)
CDA 2013 (most recent)	IGT
	FPG: < 140 mg/dL and 2h-PG: 140-199 mg/dL
	IFG
	FPG :110-125 mg/dL
	HbA1c (definition of prediabetes)
	6.0 – 6.4%

Abbreviations: NDDG, National Diabetes Data Group; WHO, World Health Organization; ADA, American Diabetes Association; CDA, Canadian Diabetes Association; IFG, impaired fasting glucose; IGT, impaired glucose tolerance; FPG, fasting plasma glucose; 2h-PG; 2-h plasma glucose; HbA1c, Hemoglobin A1c.

However, the term prediabetes itself has been criticized due to the following reasons: (1) many individuals with prediabetes do not progress to T2DM, (2) the term may imply that no intervention is necessary as no disease is present, and (3) diabetes risk does not necessarily differ between individuals with prediabetes and those with a combination of other diabetes risk factors [16]. Therefore, the WHO use the term, Intermediate Hyperglycaemia, and an International Expert Committee, convened by the ADA, use the term, High Risk State of Developing Diabetes, rather than 'prediabetes' [10, 17]. For brevity, we use the term prediabetes in this review to refer to IFG, IGT, and high risk based on HbA1c levels.

2. Prevalence of Prediabetes

The prevalence estimates of prediabetes vary according to the definition of prediabetes among the studies, the type and combination of glycemic tests in use, and the demographic characteristics of the population being measured [18]. In addition, the reproducibility of prediabetes (~50%) is lower than that for T2DM (>70%) and the alternative definitions based on IFG, IGT, and HbA1c define overlapping prediabetic groups with single or combined abnormalities [19].

In the US, in individuals aged ≥ 12 years, the age-adjusted prevalence of prediabetes (FPG 100–125 mg/dL or HbA1c 5.7%–6.4%) increased from 27.4% in 1999–2002 to 34.1% in 2007–2010. If analysis was limited to individuals aged ≥ 18 years, the prevalence increased from 29.2% to 36.2% [20]. In England, the prevalence of prediabetes (HbA1c 5.7%–6.4%) in individuals aged ≥ 16 increased from 11.6% to 35.3% from 2003 to 2011. By 2011, 50.6% of the English population who had a body mass index (BMI) >25 and were ≥40 years of age, had prediabetes [21]. In 2011, the proportion of adults with prediabetes in England was comparable to the proportion of affected individuals in the US [20, 21]. In the Chinese population aged ≥ 18, the 2010 prevalence estimate of prediabetes was even higher at 50.1%, may be due to the combination of the three glycemic indices used (FPG 100–125 mg/dL, 2h-PG 140–199 mg/dL, or HbA1c 5.7–6.4%) for defining prediabetes [22]. In a Japanese working population (47,172 men and 8,280 women; aged, 20–69 years), the prevalence of prediabetes (FPG 110–125 mg/dL or HbA1c 6.0%–6.4%) was reported as 14.1% in men and 9.2% in women [23].

Using the 2005–2008 National Health and Nutrition Examination Surveys, James et al. investigated 3,627 individuals aged ≥18 years without diabetes, and reported that the crude prevalence of prediabetes was 14.2% for HbA1c (5.7%–6.4%), 26.2% for FPG_{low} (100–125 mg/dL), 7.0% for FPG_{high} (110–125 mg/dL), and 13.7% for 2h-PG (140–199 mg/dL) [18]. Although the prevalence of prediabetes defined using HbA1c and FPG_{low} was similar for men and women, the prevalence of prediabetes defined using FPG_{high} was approximately 1.7 times higher among men than women. Furthermore, when HbA1c was used, age-adjusted prevalence among non-Hispanic blacks was almost twice that of non-Hispanic whites and Mexican ethnicity [18]. The specific choice of a prediabetes measure will yield differing associations with age, sex, and race. However, a recent analysis of prospective cohort data from the Atherosclerosis Risk in Communities Study did not support the use of race-specific thresholds in HbA1c levels for identifying individuals at risk for T2DM [24].

3. Insulin Secretion and Resistance in Prediabetes

The San Antonio Metabolism (SAM) study [25] and the Veterans Administration Genetic Epidemiology Study [26] have shown a progressive decline in pancreatic β-cell function in prediabetic individuals. The SAM study has demonstrated that when the 2h-PG level during an OGTT was 180–190 mg/dL, β-cell function had already declined by 75%– 80% [25].

IGT and IFG are reported to be metabolically distinct entities that affect different subpopulations, albeit with some degree of overlap [27, 28]. Out of the individuals who had IFG and/or IGT, 16% had both, 23% had IFG alone, and 60% had IGT alone, with significant age and gender differences among the glucose intolerance categories. The prevalence of IFG tends to plateau in middle age, whereas the prevalence of IGT rises into old age. IFG is substantially more common among men and IGT slightly more common among women [27, 28].

The pattern of insulin secretion also differs between IGT and IFG. Individuals with IGT have moderate to severe muscle insulin resistance and normal to slightly decreased hepatic insulin sensitivity. They are characterized by defects in both early- (0–30 min) and late-phase (60–120 min) insulin secretion in an OGTT. On the other hand, individuals with IFG have moderate hepatic insulin resistance with normal muscle insulin sensitivity and decreased basal and early-phase of insulin secretion. The combination of hepatic insulin resistance and defective insulin secretion in IFG results in excessive fasting hepatic glucose production accounting for fasting hyperglycemia. The impairment in early insulin response in combination with hepatic insulin resistance results in the excessive early rise of plasma glucose in the first hour of the OGTT.

However, the preservation of late insulin secretion combined with normal muscle insulin sensitivity allows glucose levels to return to the preload value in IFG [29].

4. Impact of Triglycerides on Insulin Secretion on Prediabetes

T2DM is known to be associated with plasma lipid and lipoprotein abnormalities, including reduced high-density lipoprotein cholesterol (HDL-C) and elevated triglycerides (TG) [30]. These atherogenic lipid abnormalities often precede T2DM by several years, indicating that altered lipoprotein metabolism is an early event in the development of β-cell dysfunction. Among prediabetic individuals, hypertriglyceridemia is demonstrated as a predictor of T2DM progression [31].

One of the empirical indices that measures β-cell function, the insulinogenic index (Δinsulin/Δglucose [0–30 min]), is a surrogate measure of early-phase insulin secretion [26]. In 2014, we reported the relationship between TG, HDL-C, TG/HDL-C ratio, and early-phase insulin secretion in normoglycemic and prediabetic individuals [32]. In this study, we investigated 663 Japanese individuals with either normal glucose tolerance (NGT; n = 341), isolated impaired fasting glucose (i-IFG; n = 211), isolated impaired glucose tolerance (i-IGT; n = 71), or combined IFG and IGT (IFG + IGT; n = 40). In prediabetic individuals (i-IFG, i-IGT, and IFG + IGT), linear regression analyses revealed that the insulinogenic index was positively correlated with HDL-C levels. Moreover, in individuals with i-IGT and IFG + IGT, but not with i-IFG, the insulinogenic index was negatively correlated with the log-transformed TG and TG/HDL-C ratio. Our results suggest that early-phase insulin secretion is affected by HDL-C and TG in prediabetic individuals. Furthermore, we retrospectively investigated the relationship between TG levels and the rate of change in early-phase insulin secretion in prediabetic individuals [33]. To evaluate insulin secretion, 50 prediabetic individuals underwent a 75 g-OGTT at the beginning of the study (baseline), and they were re-examined after a 2 year interval. The results showed that the rate of change in the insulinogenic index was negatively correlated with log-transformed baseline TG levels, but not with baseline HDL-C levels. Multiple linear regression analysis confirmed that the rate of change in the insulinogenic index was negatively correlated with the log-transformed baseline TG levels (Figure 1). Because fasting TG $\geq$ 150 mg/dL is an accepted criterion for identifying individuals at high risk of T2DM [34], the regression line in Figure 1 indicates that a log-transformed TG level of 2.17 (equivalent to a TG level of 150 mg/dL) may not change the insulinogenic index.

These results indicate that TG levels among prediabetic individuals should be carefully monitored and prospective studies are required to confirm our findings.

5. Impact of Uric Acid on Insulin Secretion in Normal Glucose Tolerance

Elevated serum uric acid (SUA) is an independent predictor of vascular complications and mortality in T2DM [35] and is associated with excess risk for development of T2DM [36, 37]. A recent study showed that SUA levels were strongly associated with 1h-PG levels in hypertensive individuals with normal glucose tolerance (NGT) [38], and were positively correlated with 2h-PG levels in nondiabetic individuals [39]. In a recent meta-analysis of 11 studies, SUA levels were closely associated with an increased risk of incidence of T2DM, indicating a 17 % increment in the risk of T2DM per 1 mg/dL increase in SUA levels [40].

In 2014, we investigated the relationship between SUA concentrations and early-phase insulin secretion following a 75 g-OGTT in Japanese individuals with NGT (354 men and 216 women, aged 50.5 ± 8.9 years and 52.6 ± 7.3 years, respectively). In women, multivariate linear regression analysis revealed that SUA levels were the major predictors of early-phase insulin secretion. However, in men, SUA levels did not correlate with insulin secretion [41]. These results support the hypothesis that hyperuricemia may have a direct negative effect on pancreatic β-cells inwomen with NGT.

The Kailuan Study is a 4-year prospective cohort study conducted in Chinese individuals (41,350 men and 13,328 women) without T2DM and IFG (FPG = 100–125 mg/dL). Thisprospective study suggests that there is a higher risk of developing IFG associated with low or high SUA concentrations in men. On the other hand, there is no significant correlation between developing IFG and SUA concentrations in women [42]. A study based on data from a health census survey of the Japanese population showed that elevated SUA is an independent risk factor of IFG (FPG=110–125 mg/dL) only for women.

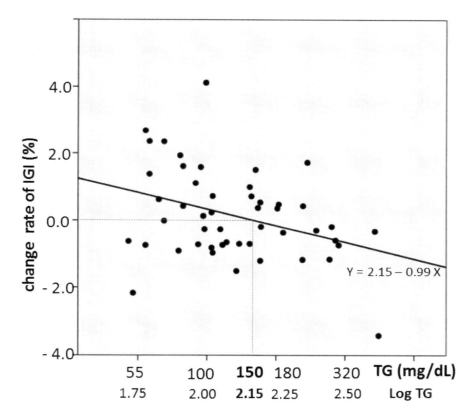

Figure 1. Correlations between the rate of change of insulinogenic index and baseline triglyceride levels.

Furthermore, in a community based epidemiological study among an adult Chinese nondiabetic population, Chou et al found that the extent of association of SUA levels with insulin resistance and plasma glucose levels was more in women than in men [43]. SUA can affect glucose metabolism in men and/or women differentially and the mechanisms of this difference requires further study.

6. Risk of Cardiovascular Disease in Prediabetes

The collaborative Diabetes in Europe: Classification and Diagnostic Criteria (DECODE) study confirmed that asymptomatic hyperglycemia is associated with an increased risk of premature mortality and cardiovascular disease (CVD) [44]. In particular, there was a graded relationship between mortality and 2h-PG. Moreover, the relationship between 2h-PG and risk of CVD is linear, while that between FPG and the risk of CVD may be nonlinear [45, 46]. Compared with FPG of 70–100 mg/dL, the relative risk (RR) for CVD were 1.07 for FPG < 70 mg/dL; 1.11 for FPG = 100–110 mg/dL; and 1.17 for FPG = 110–126 mg/dL [46].

Studies that were based on the WHO criteria of IGT (FPG < 140 mg/dL and 2h-PG = 140–199 < 200 mg/dL) reported an approximate doubling of risk for CVD among participants with IGT [47, 48]. However, other studies using the same WHO classification found estimates of RR approximately 1.15–1.22 [49, 50]. A recent meta-analysis of 8 studies examining the impact of IGT (2h-PG = 140–199 mg/dL) on CVD showed an overall estimate of RR was 1.24 (95% CI: 1.11–1.38). After adjusting for age, smoking status, blood pressure, and lipids, the estimate of RR was 1.20 (95% CI: 1.06–1.35) [51]. Some previous studies suggested that the estimated RR of CVD mortality was greater among women with borderline diabetes than men. However, this meta-analysis did not support a significant gender difference in the estimates of RR. The finding from the DECODE study also showed that the RRs for CVD among participants with 2h-PG abnormalities corresponding to IGT were very similar for men and women [45].

Because previous studies were based on a single determination of glycemic status at baseline, the question arises as to whether the risk for developing CVD is confined to people with IGT who develop T2DM or whether the risk is still increased among people with IGT even if they never develop T2DM. In a recent prospective study with systematically repeated assessment of glycemic values during the follow-up phase among IGT (defined as FPG < 140 mg/dL and 2h-PG = 140–199 mg/dL), an increased level of the current 2h-PG, recorded as the updated (last) value of yearly estimates of 2 h-PG during follow-up, was related to increased risk of CVD independent of other glycemic markers such as FPG, 1 h-PG, and HbA1c. The current level of 2 h-PG at the last measurement before the CVD event showed the highest risk increase for CVD (119%) when the various glucose measures were standardized to 1 SD increment [52]. This prospective study supports the current value of 2 h-PG as the strongest predictor for CVD and may be a useful tool in screening for IGT and when monitoring the glycemic control in individuals with IGT.

Compared with IGT, the exact magnitude of the risk for CVD associated with IFG remains opaque. There are sparse reports on the association of IFG with the development of CVD [53, 54], but data regarding the extent to which risk for CVD is increased, are inconclusive [51, 55]. The Funagata Diabetes Study which was conducted in Japanese populations showed the cumulative survival rate of IFG (FPG = 110–125 mg/ dL) from CVD was 0.977, but not significantly lower than that of NGT (0.985) at the end of seven observed years. The Cox's hazard ratio of IFG to NGT on CVD mortality was 1.14 (95% CI: 0.35–3.73), which was also not significant [48]. In other studies involving Asian population, when IFG was defined as 110–125 mg/dL, it was associated with a significant increase in CVD mortality, whereas when IFG was defined as 100–125 mg/dL mortality risks diminished substantially [56]. Furthermore, this study found an overall J-shaped relationship between all-cause mortality and levels of FPG, with significant increases in mortality, starting at $\geq$110 mg/dL as well as $\leq$75 mg/dL. This finding of a J-shaped relationship with increased mortality risk at FBG < 75 mg/dL may have important implications in the clinical management of IFG.

A recent meta-analysis including 29,893 participants showed that the fixed-effects summary estimates of RR for CVD was 1.37 (95% CI: 1.21–1.55) in IFG$_{high}$ (PFG=110–125 mg/dL) and 1.19 (95% CI: 1.08–1.32) in IFG$_{low}$ individuals (FPG=100–125 mg/dL) [51]. The analysis indicates that the estimated RR for CVD in IFG ranges from approximately 1.12–1.37, depending on the set of studies included in a particular analysis. Furthermore, the increased risk of IFG remained significantly elevated, even after risk factors for CVD were adjusted. In other words, IFG is capable of independently predicting the future mortality, and identifying individuals with IFG is not an incidental or benign finding.

These days, there is no compelling evidence to suggest that the estimated RR for IGT is greater than that for IFG. However, beyond the differences existing in establishing IFG (the normal limit for FPG) depending on the institution, the FPG may have a direct relationship with increased risk for CVD. There is a growing need to emphasize early and vigilant risk factor management in prediabetic individuals to reduce their CVD morbidity and mortality.

7. Progression from NGT
to Prediabetes and T2DM

Around 5%–10% of people with prediabetes are diagnosed with T2DM every year. The natural history of both IFG and IGT is variable, with 25% progressing to T2DM, 50% remaining in their abnormal glycemic state, and 25% reverting to NGT over an observational period of 3–5 years [57, 58]. In an evaluation of 6 prospective studies of different populations, the combined incidence rate of T2DM was 57.2 per 1,000 patient-years in individuals with IGT [59]. On the other hand, there is controversy about the progression of T2DM in IFG, ranging from 9.0%–30.0% for periods from 5–10 years of evolution [6, 60]. The combination of increasing FPG and 2-h PG confers greater risk for T2DM than either in isolation; the odds ratios for T2DM are reported as 10.1, 10.9, and 39.5 for those having IFG, IGT, and combined IFG and IGT, respectively [6]. Therefore, regression from IFG/IGT to isolated IFG or isolated IGT may also decrease the risk of T2DM. For comparison, women with gestational diabetes have been suggested as having a 20%–60% risk of developing diabetes 5–10 years after pregnancy. In a recent meta-analysis of 20 studies, 13% of mothers with gestational diabetes developed diabetes after pregnancy compared to 1% of mothers without gestational diabetes [61].

The risk factors for T2DM are of three types: modifiable risk factors that include obesity, hypertension, lipid disorders, hyperuricemia, unhealthy diet, and low physical activity; non-modifiable risk factors that include age, family history of T2DM, ethnicity, and low-birth weight; and environmental risk factors that include low socioeconomic status, cultural constraints, religious practices, and distress. The impact on development of T2DM due to risk factors is exerted through a combinatorial interplay of risk factors from all of the aforementioned three types. However, the predisposing factors for prediabetes have not yet been well established. More precisely, the significance of attenuated glucose-stimulated insulin secretion, insulin sensitivity, and β-cell function for the deterioration of glucose metabolism from NGT to IFG and/or IGT has not been fully clarified [62-65]. Accurate prediction of deteriorating glucose regulation in individuals with NGT is mandatory for intervention aiming at halting the development of prediabetes.

In obese Pima Indians, Weyer et al. reported that low glucose-stimulated insulin secretion and low insulin sensitivity, but not male gender and increased BMI, were risk factors for development from NGT to IGT [66]. In addition to the above risk factors, in mildly overweight Europids, positive family history of T2DM was also a risk factor for deteriorating glucose tolerance. Five-year follow-up data from a Danish population showed that plasma glucose and insulin levels at baseline were higher, and insulin sensitivity and early-phase insulin secretion were lower in individuals who progressed to prediabetes (IFG, IGT, or IFG/IGT) than in those who maintained NGT status. During the 5-year follow-up period, individuals developing IFG experienced a significant decline only in insulin sensitivity, whereas individuals developing IGT experienced significant declines in insulin sensitivity and early-phase insulin secretion [64]. Recently, a longitudinal analysis of a middle-aged Japanese cohort with NGT reported that attenuated β-cell function was an independent risk factor for developing IFG, and lower insulin sensitivity was an additional risk for developing IGT. Furthermore, this study showed that positive family history was a strong risk factor only for IGT, whereas male gender and elevated BMI and plasma glucose levels (FPG or 2h-PG) were common risk factors for both IGT and IFG [67]. These studies support the notion that the prediabetic states of IFG and IGT may have different etiological and pathophysiological origins, which may have implications on the prevention and treatment of the T2DM that succeeds them.

8. Predictor for Regression from Prediabetes to NGT

Previous studies have demonstrated reductions between 25%–72% in the incidence of T2DM over 2.4–6 year lifestyle intervention periods, with most participants remaining prediabetic. The Diabetes Prevention Program (DPP) Research Group randomized 3,234 individuals with IFG and IGT to receive placebo, metformin, or a lifestyle-intervention program. After an average of 2.8 years, the incidence of T2DM was 11.0, 7.8, and 4.8 cases per 100 person-years, respectively [4]. Less often discussed are the 20%–50% of participants that not only did not progress, but in fact, reverted to NGT (FPG < 100 mg/dL and 2h-PG < 140 mg/dL) [4, 68-70]. These results indicate prediabetes can convert back to NGT. Although risk factors for T2DM are well established, far less is known about factors associated with reversal of the process.

In 2009, Perreault et al. reported a post-hoc analysis from the DPP examining predictors of regression from prediabetes to NGT over 3-year follow-up. This analysis revealed that, in addition to intensive lifestyle modification, weight loss had significant and independent effects on regression. Interestingly, intensive lifestyle modification predicted regression to NGR independent of weight loss in this study. Furthermore, younger age, lower baseline FPG and 2-h PG, and greater insulin secretion predicted regression to NGT. On the other hand, a non-significant trend for regression was observed for metformin, male gender, and insulin sensitivity [71]. Some of the aforementioned factors governing the return to NGT are modifiable, and others are not. Therefore, establishing healthy habits early in life, before age-related changes occur, may be the best strategy for regression from prediabetes to NGT.

9. Intervention to Prevent Progression to Prediabetes

Although many drugs are available and recommended for the management of T2DM, the guidelines from different associations only recommend lifestyle modifications for prediabetes [72, 73]. Though prediabetes is regarded as a precursor stage of T2DM, which does not require active management, apart from a strict control in diet and adequate exercise, this view has been challenged ever since voglibose has been approved for the management of IGT in Japan [74]. A double-blind, placebo-controlled clinical trial carried out in a Japanese IGT population confirmed a significant effect of voglibose on the primary prevention of T2DM compared with the placebo [75]. Furthermore, among Japanese individuals with IGT, voglibose with standard care of diet and exercise resulted in cost-saving, as well as prolongation of life expectancy, compared with standard care alone [76]. Other anti-diabetic agents may also have a beneficial effect on prevention of prediabetes. The GLP-1 analogues (exenatide and liraglutide) were both found to produce sustained weight loss among obese individuals, and were associated with increased reversion from prediabetes to normoglycaemia over 1–2 years follow-up [77, 78]. In addition, a recently published meta-analysis concluded that the therapy of prediabetic individuals with thiazolidinediones and α-glucosidase inhibitors was associated with increased odds of regression to NGT than with controls [79]. In contrast, a double-blind, randomized clinical trial with 9,306 participants having IGT showed that assignment to nateglinide for 5-years did not reduce the incidence of T2DM [80].

Weight loss appears to be the most important component of intensive lifestyle intervention predicting regression, with every 1 kg lost associated with a 16% reduction in risk for T2DM [81]. Recent data suggest that lifestyle interventions to prevent T2DM may overcome the genetic risk of T2DM [82]. This information may be helpful to parents of children with a strong family history of T2DM. The DPP, a randomized controlled clinical trial which predominantly included obese, middle aged individuals with IGT demonstrated that compared with the placebo intervention, the intensive lifestyle intervention reduced the incidence of T2DM by 58%, and the metformin intervention reduced the incidence of T2DM by 31% over 2.8 years [4]. This study indicates improved insulin secretion relative to insulin sensitivity after 1 year of intensive lifestyle intervention. The Diabetes Prevention Program Outcomes Study (DPPOS) has followed the participants for an additional 7-years during which participants in lifestyle- and metformin-intervention groups were encouraged to continue those interventions, and all participants were offered a group-lifestyle intervention [83]. The incidence of T2DM during the 10-year average follow-up after randomization was reduced by 34% in those initially randomized to lifestyle and 18% in those initially randomized to metformin compared with placebo [83]. Results from DPPOS would contend that the strategy is important as long as the intervention is early (individual has been diagnosed with prediabetes) and can restore NGT, even if transiently. Furthermore, over 10-years, from a tax-payers perspective, lifestyle was cost-effective and metformin was marginally cost-saving compared with placebo [84]. Investment in lifestyle and metformin interventions for prevention of T2DM in high-risk adults may be cost-effective.

Conclusion

There is a global epidemic of prediabetes. Prediabetes is associated with an increased risk of developing T2DM and CVD. Lifestyle intervention and pharmacological intervention treatment for prediabetes prevent the onset of overt T2DM. Furthermore, interventions for prediabetes can return individuals to NGT. Therefore, true prevention for T2DM may reside in the restoration to NGT rather than in the maintenance of a high-risk state. Framing prediabetes as a preventable disease and not a risk or a 'pre' stage for T2DM is required to facilitate early management. Development of clinical guidelines on how to identify and manage prediabetic individuals is essential. In addition, development of a low-cost, easily accessible lifestyle management program is required for the hundreds of thousands of individuals with prediabetes.

Strategies targeting interventions aimed at the entire population at risk of prediabetes can make health care more affordable, mitigate against a preventable disease, and save lives.

Acknowledgments

The author would like to acknowledge the efforts of Jun Shimizu. There are no relationships with industry.

References

[1]   Yoon, K. H., Lee, J. H., Kim, J. W., Cho, J. H., Choi, Y. H., Ko, S. H., Zimmet, P., Son, H. Y. Epidemic obesity and type 2 diabetes in Asia. *Lancet* 2006; 368:1681-1688.

[2]   Amos, A. F., McCarty, D. J., Zimmet, P. The rising global burden of diabetes and its complications: estimates and projections to the year 2010. *Diabetic medicine: a journal of the British Diabetic Association* 1997; 14 Suppl. 5:S1-85.

[3]   Tuomilehto, J., Lindstrom, J., Eriksson, J. G., Valle, T. T., Hamalainen, H., Ilanne-Parikka, P., Keinanen-Kiukaanniemi, S., Laakso, M., Louheranta, A., Rastas, M., et al. Prevention of type 2 diabetes mellitus by changes in lifestyle among subjects with impaired glucose tolerance. *The New England journal of medicine* 2001; 344:1343-1350.

[4]   Knowler, W. C., Barrett-Connor, E., Fowler, S. E., Hamman, R. F., Lachin, J. M., Walker, E. A., Nathan, D. M. Reduction in the incidence of type 2 diabetes with lifestyle intervention or metformin. *The New England journal of medicine* 2002; 346:393-403.

[5]   Vendrame, F., Gottlieb, P. A. Prediabetes: prediction and prevention trials. *Endocrinology and metabolism clinics of North America* 2004; 33: 75-92, ix.

[6]   de Vegt, F., Dekker, J. M., Jager, A., Hienkens, E., Kostense, P. J., Stehouwer, C. D., Nijpels, G., Bouter, L. M., Heine, R. J. Relation of impaired fasting and postload glucose with incident type 2 diabetes in a Dutch population: The Hoorn Study. *JAMA* 2001; 285:2109-2113.

[7] Gagliardino, J. J. Physiological endocrine control of energy homeostasis and postprandial blood glucose levels. *European review for medical and pharmacological sciences* 2005; 9:75-92.

[8] Classification and diagnosis of diabetes mellitus and other categories of glucose intolerance. National Diabetes Data Group. *Diabetes* 1979; 28: 1039-1057.

[9] Report of the Expert Committee on the Diagnosis and Classification of Diabetes Mellitus. *Diabetes care* 1997; 20:1183-1197.

[10] World Health Organization and International Diabetes Federation. *Definition and diagnosis of diabetes mellitus and intermediate hyperglycaemia: report of a WHO/IDF consultation.* Geneva. World Health Organization 2006.

[11] Report of the expert committee on the diagnosis and classification of diabetes mellitus. *Diabetes care* 2003; 26 Suppl. 1:S5-20.

[12] Zhang, X., Gregg, E. W., Williamson, D. F., Barker, L. E., Thomas, W., Bullard, K. M., Imperatore, G., Williams, D. E., Albright, A. L. A1C level and future risk of diabetes: a systematic review. *Diabetes care* 2010; 33:1665-1673.

[13] Standards of medical care in diabetes--2014. *Diabetes care* 2014; 37 Suppl. 1:S14-80.

[14] Goldenberg, R., Punthakee, Z. Definition, classification and diagnosis of diabetes, prediabetes and metabolic syndrome. *Canadian journal of diabetes* 2013; 37 Suppl. 1:S8-11.

[15] Diagnosis and classification of diabetes mellitus. *Diabetes care* 2012; 35 Suppl. 1:S64-71.

[16] Tabak, A. G., Herder, C., Rathmann, W., Brunner, E. J., Kivimaki, M. Prediabetes: a high-risk state for diabetes development. *Lancet* 2012; 379:2279-2290.

[17] International Expert Committee report on the role of the A1C assay in the diagnosis of diabetes. *Diabetes care* 2009; 32:1327-1334.

[18] James, C., Bullard, K. M., Rolka, D. B., Geiss, L. S., Williams, D. E., Cowie, C. C., Albright, A., Gregg, E. W. Implications of alternative definitions of prediabetes for prevalence in US adults. *Diabetes care* 2011; 34:387-391.

[19] Balion, C. M., Raina, P. S., Gerstein, H. C., Santaguida, P. L., Morrison, K. M., Booker, L., Hunt, D. L. Reproducibility of impaired glucose tolerance (IGT) and impaired fasting glucose (IFG) classification: a systematic review. *Clinical chemistry and laboratory medicine: CCLM / FESCC* 2007; 45:1180-1185.

[20] Bullard, K. M., Saydah, S. H., Imperatore, G., Cowie, C. C., Gregg, E.
      W., Geiss, L. S., Cheng, Y. J., Rolka, D. B., Williams, D. E., Caspersen,
      C. J. Secular changes in US Prediabetes prevalence defined by
      hemoglobin A1c and fasting plasma glucose: National Health and
      Nutrition Examination Surveys, 1999-2010. *Diabetes care* 2013; 36:
      2286-2293.
[21] Mainous, A. G., 3rd, Tanner, R. J., Baker, R., Zayas, C. E., Harle, C. A.
      Prevalence of prediabetes in England from 2003 to 2011: population-
      based, cross-sectional study. *BMJ open* 2014; 4:e005002.
[22] Xu, Y., Wang, L., He, J., Bi, Y., Li, M., Wang, T., Jiang, Y., Dai, M.,
      Lu, J., Xu, M., et al. Prevalence and control of diabetes in Chinese
      adults. *JAMA* 2013; 310:948-959.
[23] Uehara, A., Kurotani, K., Kochi, T., Kuwahara, K., Eguchi, M., Imai, T.,
      Nishihara, A., Tomita, K., Yamamoto, M., Kuroda, R., et al. Prevalence
      of diabetes and pre-diabetes among workers: Japan Epidemiology
      Collaboration on Occupational Health Study. *Diabetes research and
      clinical practice* 2014; 106:118-127.
[24] Selvin, E., Steffes, M. W., Zhu, H., Matsushita, K., Wagenknecht, L.,
      Pankow, J., Coresh, J., Brancati, F. L. Glycated hemoglobin, diabetes,
      and cardiovascular risk in nondiabetic adults. *The New England journal
      of medicine* 2010; 362:800-811.
[25] Gastaldelli, A., Ferrannini, E., Miyazaki, Y., Matsuda, M., DeFronzo, R.
      A. Beta-cell dysfunction and glucose intolerance: results from the San
      Antonio metabolism (SAM) study. *Diabetologia* 2004; 47:31-39.
[26] Abdul-Ghani, M. A., Tripathy, D., DeFronzo, R. A. Contributions of
      beta-cell dysfunction and insulin resistance to the pathogenesis of
      impaired glucose tolerance and impaired fasting glucose. *Diabetes care*
      2006; 29:1130-1139.
[27] Unwin, N., Shaw, J., Zimmet, P., Alberti, K. G. Impaired glucose
      tolerance and impaired fasting glycaemia: the current status on definition
      and intervention. *Diabetic medicine: a journal of the British Diabetic
      Association* 2002; 19:708-723.
[28] Williams, J. W., Zimmet, P. Z., Shaw, J. E., de Courten, M. P.,
      Cameron, A. J., Chitson, P., Tuomilehto, J., Alberti, K. G. Gender
      differences in the prevalence of impaired fasting glycaemia and impaired
      glucose tolerance in Mauritius. Does sex matter? *Diabetic medicine: a
      journal of the British Diabetic Association* 2003; 20:915-920.
[29] Nathan, D. M., Davidson, M. B., DeFronzo, R. A., Heine, R. J., Henry,
      R. R., Pratley, R., Zinman, B. Impaired fasting glucose and impaired

glucose tolerance: implications for care. *Diabetes care* 2007; 30:753-759.

[30] Haffner, S. M. Management of dyslipidemia in adults with diabetes. *Diabetes care* 2003; 26 Suppl. 1:S83-86.

[31] Rasmussen, S. S., Glumer, C., Sandbaek, A., Lauritzen, T., Borch-Johnsen, K. Determinants of progression from impaired fasting glucose and impaired glucose tolerance to diabetes in a high-risk screened population: 3 year follow-up in the ADDITION study, Denmark. *Diabetologia* 2008; 51:249-257.

[32] Shimodaira, M., Niwa, T., Nakajima, K., Kobayashi, M., Hanyu, N., Nakayama, T. Impact of serum triglyceride and high density lipoprotein cholesterol levels on early-phase insulin secretion in normoglycemic and prediabetic subjects. *Diabetes and metabolism journal* 2014; 38:294-301.

[33] Shimodaira, M., Niwa, T., Nakajima, K., Kobayashi, M., Hanyu, N., Nakayama, T. Serum Triglyceride Levels Correlated with the Rate of Change in Insulin Secretion Over Two Years in Prediabetic Subjects. *Annals of nutrition and metabolism* 2014; 64:38-43.

[34] Executive Summary of The Third Report of The National Cholesterol Education Program (NCEP) Expert Panel on Detection, Evaluation, And Treatment of High Blood Cholesterol In Adults (Adult Treatment Panel III). *JAMA* 2001; 285:2486-2497.

[35] Xu, Y., Zhu, J., Gao, L., Liu, Y., Shen, J., Shen, C., Matfin, G., Wu, X. Hyperuricemia as an independent predictor of vascular complications and mortality in type 2 diabetes patients: a meta-analysis. *PLoS ONE* 2013; 8:e78206.

[36] Krishnan, E., Akhras, K. S., Sharma, H., Marynchenko, M., Wu, E. Q., Tawk, R., Liu, J., Shi, L. Relative and attributable diabetes risk associated with hyperuricemia in US veterans with gout. *QJM: monthly journal of the Association of Physicians* 2013; 106:721-729.

[37] Krishnan, E., Pandya, B. J., Chung, L., Hariri, A., Dabbous, O. Hyperuricemia in young adults and risk of insulin resistance, prediabetes, and diabetes: a 15-year follow-up study. *American journal of epidemiology* 2012; 176:108-116.

[38] Perticone, F., Sciacqua, A., Perticone, M., Arturi, F., Scarpino, P. E., Quero, M., Sesti, G. Serum uric acid and 1-h postload glucose in essential hypertension. *Diabetes care* 2012; 35:153-157.

[39] Hodge, A. M., Boyko, E. J., de Courten, M., Zimmet, P. Z., Chitson, P., Tuomilehto, J., Alberti, K. G. Leptin and other components of the

Metabolic Syndrome in Mauritius--a factor analysis. *International journal of obesity and related metabolic disorders: journal of the International Association for the Study of Obesity* 2001; 25:126-131.

[40] Kodama, S., Saito, K., Yachi, Y., Asumi, M., Sugawara, A., Totsuka, K., Saito, A., Sone, H. Association between serum uric acid and development of type 2 diabetes. *Diabetes care* 2009; 32:1737-1742.

[41] Shimodaira, M., Niwa, T., Nakajima, K., Kobayashi, M., Hanyu, N., Nakayama, T. The Relationship Between Serum Uric Acid Levels and beta-Cell Functions in Nondiabetic Subjects. *Hormone and metabolic research = Hormon- und Stoffwechselforschung = Hormones et metabolisme* 2014; 46:950-954.

[42] Liu, Y., Jin, C., Xing, A., Liu, X., Chen, S., Li, D., Feng, P., Liu, J., Li, Z., Wu, S. Serum uric acid levels and the risk of impaired fasting glucose: a prospective study in adults of north China. *PLoS ONE* 2013; 8:e84712.

[43] Chou, P., Lin, K. C., Lin, H. Y., Tsai, S. T. Gender differences in the relationships of serum uric acid with fasting serum insulin and plasma glucose in patients without diabetes. *The Journal of rheumatology* 2001; 28:571-576.

[44] Glucose tolerance and mortality: comparison of WHO and American Diabetes Association diagnostic criteria. The DECODE study group. European Diabetes Epidemiology Group. Diabetes Epidemiology: Collaborative analysis Of Diagnostic criteria in Europe. *Lancet* 1999; 354:617-621.

[45] Glucose tolerance and cardiovascular mortality: comparison of fasting and 2-hour diagnostic criteria. *Archives of internal medicine* 2001; 161: 397-405.

[46] Sarwar, N., Gao, P., Seshasai, S. R., Gobin, R., Kaptoge, S., Di Angelantonio, E., Ingelsson, E., Lawlor, D. A., Selvin, E., Stampfer, M., et al. Diabetes mellitus, fasting blood glucose concentration, and risk of vascular disease: a collaborative meta-analysis of 102 prospective studies. *Lancet* 2010; 375:2215-2222.

[47] Fujishima, M., Kiyohara, Y., Kato, I., Ohmura, T., Iwamoto, H., Nakayama, K., Ohmori, S., Yoshitake, T. Diabetes and cardiovascular disease in a prospective population survey in Japan: The Hisayama Study. *Diabetes* 1996; 45 Suppl. 3:S14-16.

[48] Tominaga, M., Eguchi, H., Manaka, H., Igarashi, K., Kato, T., Sekikawa, A. Impaired glucose tolerance is a risk factor for

cardiovascular disease, but not impaired fasting glucose. The Funagata Diabetes Study. *Diabetes care* 1999; 22:920-924.

[49] Barzilay, J. I., Spiekerman, C. F., Wahl, P. W., Kuller, L. H., Cushman, M., Furberg, C. D., Dobs, A., Polak, J. F., Savage, P. J. Cardiovascular disease in older adults with glucose disorders: comparison of American Diabetes Association criteria for diabetes mellitus with WHO criteria. *Lancet* 1999; 354:622-625.

[50] de Vegt, F., Dekker, J. M., Ruhe, H. G., Stehouwer, C. D., Nijpels, G., Bouter, L. M., Heine, R. J. Hyperglycaemia is associated with all-cause and cardiovascular mortality in the Hoorn population: the Hoorn Study. *Diabetologia* 1999; 42:926-931.

[51] Ford, E. S., Zhao, G., Li, C. Pre-diabetes and the risk for cardiovascular disease: a systematic review of the evidence. *Journal of the American College of Cardiology* 2010; 55:1310-1317.

[52] Lind, M., Tuomilehto, J., Uusitupa, M., Nerman, O., Eriksson, J., Ilanne-Parikka, P., Keinanen-Kiukaanniemi, S., Peltonen, M., Pivodic, A., Lindstrom, J. The association between HbA1c, fasting glucose, 1-hour glucose and 2-hour glucose during an oral glucose tolerance test and cardiovascular disease in individuals with elevated risk for diabetes. *PLoS ONE* 2014; 9:e109506.

[53] Milman, S., Crandall, J. P. Mechanisms of vascular complications in prediabetes. *The Medical clinics of North America* 2011; 95:309-325, vii.

[54] Moutzouri, E., Tsimihodimos, V., Rizos, E., Elisaf, M. Prediabetes: to treat or not to treat? *European journal of pharmacology* 2011; 672:9-19.

[55] Levitan, E. B., Song, Y., Ford, E. S., Liu, S. Is nondiabetic hyperglycemia a risk factor for cardiovascular disease? A meta-analysis of prospective studies. *Archives of internal medicine* 2004; 164:2147-2155.

[56] Wen, C. P., Cheng, T. Y., Tsai, S. P., Hsu, H. L., Wang, S. L. Increased mortality risks of pre-diabetes (impaired fasting glucose) in Taiwan. *Diabetes care* 2005; 28:2756-2761.

[57] Gabir, M. M., Hanson, R. L., Dabelea, D., Imperatore, G., Roumain, J., Bennett, P. H., Knowler, W. C. The 1997 American Diabetes Association and 1999 World Health Organization criteria for hyperglycemia in the diagnosis and prediction of diabetes. *Diabetes care* 2000; 23:1108-1112.

[58] Stern, M. P., Williams, K., Haffner, S. M. Identification of persons at high risk for type 2 diabetes mellitus: do we need the oral glucose tolerance test? *Annals of internal medicine* 2002; 136:575-581.

[59] Edelstein, S. L., Knowler, W. C., Bain, R. P., Andres, R., Barrett-Connor, E. L., Dowse, G. K., Haffner, S. M., Pettitt, D. J., Sorkin, J. D., Muller, D. C., et al. Predictors of progression from impaired glucose tolerance to NIDDM: an analysis of six prospective studies. *Diabetes* 1997; 46:701-710.

[60] Eschwege, E., Charles, M. A., Simon, D., Thibult, N., Balkau, B. Reproducibility of the diagnosis of diabetes over a 30-month follow-up: the Paris Prospective Study. *Diabetes care* 2001; 24:1941-1944.

[61] Bellamy, L., Casas, J. P., Hingorani, A. D., Williams, D. Type 2 diabetes mellitus after gestational diabetes: a systematic review and meta-analysis. *Lancet* 2009; 373:1773-1779.

[62] Goldfine, A. B., Bouche, C., Parker, R. A., Kim, C., Kerivan, A., Soeldner, J. S., Martin, B. C., Warram, J. H., Kahn, C. R. Insulin resistance is a poor predictor of type 2 diabetes in individuals with no family history of disease. *Proceedings of the National Academy of Sciences of the United States of America* 2003; 100:2724-2729.

[63] Tabak, A. G., Jokela, M., Akbaraly, T. N., Brunner, E. J., Kivimaki, M., Witte, D. R. Trajectories of glycaemia, insulin sensitivity, and insulin secretion before diagnosis of type 2 diabetes: an analysis from the Whitehall II study. *Lancet* 2009; 373:2215-2221.

[64] Faerch, K., Vaag, A., Holst, J. J., Hansen, T., Jorgensen, T., Borch-Johnsen, K. Natural history of insulin sensitivity and insulin secretion in the progression from normal glucose tolerance to impaired fasting glycemia and impaired glucose tolerance: the Inter99 study. *Diabetes care* 2009; 32:439-444.

[65] Ferrannini, E., Natali, A., Muscelli, E., Nilsson, P. M., Golay, A., Laakso, M., Beck-Nielsen, H., Mari, A. Natural history and physiological determinants of changes in glucose tolerance in a non-diabetic population: the RISC Study. *Diabetologia* 2011; 54:1507-1516.

[66] Weyer, C., Tataranni, P. A., Bogardus, C., Pratley, R. E. Insulin resistance and insulin secretory dysfunction are independent predictors of worsening of glucose tolerance during each stage of type 2 diabetes development. *Diabetes care* 2001; 24:89-94.

[67] Oka, R., Yagi, K., Hayashi, K., Kawashiri, M. A., Yamagishi, M., Yamada, M., Fumisawa, Y., Yamauchi, K., Aizawa, T. The evolution of

non-diabetic hyperglycemia: a longitudinal study. *Endocrine journal* 2014; 61:91-99.

[68] Chiasson, J. L., Josse, R. G., Gomis, R., Hanefeld, M., Karasik, A., Laakso, M. Acarbose for prevention of type 2 diabetes mellitus: the STOP-NIDDM randomised trial. *Lancet* 2002; 359:2072-2077.

[69] Eriksson, K. F., Lindgarde, F. Prevention of type 2 (non-insulin-dependent) diabetes mellitus by diet and physical exercise. The 6-year Malmo feasibility study. *Diabetologia* 1991; 34:891-898.

[70] Gerstein, H. C., Yusuf, S., Bosch, J., Pogue, J., Sheridan, P., Dinccag, N., Hanefeld, M., Hoogwerf, B., Laakso, M., Mohan, V., et al. Effect of rosiglitazone on the frequency of diabetes in patients with impaired glucose tolerance or impaired fasting glucose: a randomised controlled trial. *Lancet* 2006; 368:1096-1105.

[71] Perreault, L., Kahn, S. E., Christophi, C. A., Knowler, W. C., Hamman, R. F. Regression from pre-diabetes to normal glucose regulation in the diabetes prevention program. *Diabetes care* 2009; 32:1583-1588.

[72] Garber, A. J., Handelsman, Y., Einhorn, D., Bergman, D. A., Bloomgarden, Z. T., Fonseca, V., Garvey, W. T., Gavin, J. R., 3rd, Grunberger, G., Horton, E. S., et al. Diagnosis and management of prediabetes in the continuum of hyperglycemia: when do the risks of diabetes begin? A consensus statement from the American College of Endocrinology and the American Association of Clinical Endocrinologists. *Endocrine practice: official journal of the American College of Endocrinology and the American Association of Clinical Endocrinologists* 2008; 14:933-946.

[73] Prediabetes. Available online from http://www.diabetes.org/diabetes-basics/prevention/pre-diabetes/ Last accessed on 6th Jan. 2014.

[74] Basen®. Available online from http://www.takeda.com/news/2009/2009 1019_3730.html Last accessed on 6th Jan. 2014.

[75] Kawamori, R., Tajima, N., Iwamoto, Y., Kashiwagi, A., Shimamoto, K., Kaku, K. Voglibose for prevention of type 2 diabetes mellitus: a randomised, double-blind trial in Japanese individuals with impaired glucose tolerance. *Lancet* 2009; 373:1607-1614.

[76] Ikeda, S., Kobayashi, M., Tajima, N. Cost-effectiveness analysis of voglibose for prevention of type 2 diabetes mellitus in Japanese patients with impaired glucose tolerance. *Journal of diabetes investigation* 2010; 1:252-258.

[77] Rosenstock, J., Klaff, L. J., Schwartz, S., Northrup, J., Holcombe, J. H., Wilhelm, K., Trautmann, M. Effects of exenatide and lifestyle

modification on body weight and glucose tolerance in obese subjects with and without pre-diabetes. *Diabetes care* 2010; 33:1173-1175.

[78] Astrup, A., Rossner, S., Van Gaal, L., Rissanen, A., Niskanen, L., Al Hakim, M., Madsen, J., Rasmussen, M. F., Lean, M. E. Effects of liraglutide in the treatment of obesity: a randomised, double-blind, placebo-controlled study. *Lancet* 2009; 374:1606-1616.

[79] Phung, O. J., Baker, W. L., Tongbram, V., Bhardwaj, A., Coleman, C. I. Oral antidiabetic drugs and regression from prediabetes to normoglycemia: a meta-analysis. *The Annals of pharmacotherapy* 2012; 46:469-476.

[80] Holman, R. R., Haffner, S. M., McMurray, J. J., Bethel, M. A., Holzhauer, B., Hua, T. A., Belenkov, Y., Boolell, M., Buse, J. B., Buckley, B. M., et al. Effect of nateglinide on the incidence of diabetes and cardiovascular events. *The New England journal of medicine* 2010; 362:1463-1476.

[81] Hamman, R. F., Wing, R. R., Edelstein, S. L., Lachin, J. M., Bray, G. A., Delahanty, L., Hoskin, M., Kriska, A. M., Mayer-Davis, E. J., Pi-Sunyer, X., et al. Effect of weight loss with lifestyle intervention on risk of diabetes. *Diabetes care* 2006; 29:2102-2107.

[82] Florez, J. C. Genetic susceptibility to type 2 diabetes and implications for therapy. *Journal of diabetes science and technology* 2009; 3:690-696.

[83] Knowler, W. C., Fowler, S. E., Hamman, R. F., Christophi, C. A., Hoffman, H. J., Brenneman, A. T., Brown-Friday, J. O., Goldberg, R., Venditti, E., Nathan, D. M. 10-year follow-up of diabetes incidence and weight loss in the Diabetes Prevention Program Outcomes Study. *Lancet* 2009; 374:1677-1686.

[84] The 10-year cost-effectiveness of lifestyle intervention or metformin for diabetes prevention: an intent-to-treat analysis of the DPP/DPPOS. *Diabetes care* 2012; 35:723-730.

In: Impaired Glucose Tolerance ...
Editor: Sandra Wagner

ISBN: 978-1-63483-085-0
© 2015 Nova Science Publishers, Inc.

Chapter 2

Improvement of Estrogen Signaling Upregulates Defective Cellular Glucose Uptake and Prevents the Comorbidities of Insulin Resistance

Zsuzsanna Suba[*]
National Institute of Oncology,
Surgical and Molecular Tumor Pathology Centre,
Budapest, Hungary

Abstract

The insulin signaling pathway regulates the cellular uptake of glucose and whole-body metabolic homeostasis in mammalians. Dysregulation of insulin secretion or alterations in the transduction of insulin receptor signal are associated with self-generating, progressive insulin resistance, which predisposes patients to a variety of life threatening chronic diseases.

---

[*] Correspondent author: Prof. Dr. Zsuzsanna Suba. National Institute of Oncology, Surgical and Molecular Tumor Pathology Centre. Address: H-1122 Ráth György str. 7-9, Budapest, Hungary. Tel: 00 36 1 224 86 00; Fax: 0036 1 224 86 20; e-mail: subazdr@gmail.com.

Activation of estrogen receptor (ER) signals by estrogen has beneficial effects on glucose homeostasis and energy metabolism by several pathways. Nevertheless, certain scientific results support that an overexpression of ER isoforms or hyperestrogenism may have important implications for the development of dysmetabolism, such as metabolic syndrome, type 2 diabetes and their comorbidities. Moreover, increased estrogen synthesis is erroneously supposed to disrupt the glucose uptake in the adipose tissue mass in obese patients and is presumed to contribute to insulin resistance and the associated comorbidities. By contrast, in animal experiments, pregnancy analogue estradiol administration improves the metabolic functions and exhibits cancer preventive capacity even in insulin resistant and obese ones. In human practice, multiparity associated good estrogen signaling shows strong tumor protective effect even against the cancers of highly hormone dependent female organs including overall breast cancer, endometrial and ovarian tumors. Considering the advantageous effects of suitable estrogen signaling on insulin secretion, cellular glucose uptake and further metabolic processes, estrogen administration seems to be a new therapeutic possibility to improve insulin sensitivity in patients with metabolic syndrome and diabetes mellitus.

Introduction

Type 2 diabetes mellitus is a systemic disease based mainly on insufficient insulin action and defective cellular glucose uptake, characterized by an imbalance in energy expenditure, alterations in glucose and lipid metabolism [1] and disturbances in cell proliferation [2]. Both genetic and environmental factors play pivotal roles in the etiology of type 2 diabetes; however the main pathologic process is the insulin resistance associated disruption of glucose homeostasis [3]. The prevalence of type 2 diabetes is increasing all over the world, which may be associated with population ageing and also with the rapid spread of western lifestyle and obesity [4].

Insulin resistance may have no noticeable clinical symptoms for a long period of time; it is counteracted and hidden by an increased insulin secretion, in the course of which the ongoing process leads to diverse human diseases [5]. Earlier, cardiovascular lesions, hypertension, dyslipidemia, obesity and increased fasting glucose levels were attributed to be the complications of type 2 diabetes; however the sequence of pathologic alterations was frequently inconsistent and contradictory. Many divergent symptoms and findings seem to have a common soil, the defective glucose uptake of mammalian cells [6].

Reactive hyperinsulinemia in the first compensated phase of insulin resistance transiently maintains the serum glucose level within the normal range by the increased secretory capacity of pancreatic beta-cells [3]. Insulin also has important metabolic impacts functioning as a growth factor as well with strong mitogenic capacity, and an increased insulin level means an excessive stimulation of multiple cellular signaling cascades [7]. Hyperinsulinemia increases the synthesis and mitogenic activity of further insulin-like growth factors, such as IGF-I. At the same time, excessive insulin secretion induces a derangement of hormonal equilibrium and impaired estrogen signaling is associated with deepening metabolic disorders [8,9].

Metabolic syndrome (prediabetes) develops in the second phase of insulin resistance, when the increased insulin synthesis of pancreatic islet cells is not enough to maintain euglycemia and metabolic balance. This phase is characterized by a quartet of elevated fasting glucose, high serum triglyceride, low HDL cholesterol level and hypertension and is frequently associated with visceral obesity [10].

The metabolic syndrome is a high risk for the development of serious chronic diseases, such as cardiovascular sclerotic alterations and malignancies [6,11].

Type 2 diabetes is the uncompensated phase of insulin resistance, when the insufficient level of circulating insulin results in disturbances in cellular glucose uptake, excessive hyperglycemia, abundant formation of free radicals and glycation of proteins [12]. These noxious processes cause serious damages in all biologic structures at molecular level [13,14]. Stroke, myocardial infarct, cognitive disorders and malignant tumors are the most frequent health catastrophes associated with the terminal phase of insulin resistance.

Estrogen signaling seems to have beneficial effects on insulin secretion [15,16], cellular glucose uptake and energy metabolism [1,8,17]. Complex and multifaceted correlations between estrogen signaling and several diseases have led to the erroneous concept that estrogen levels, either low or high may lead to disorders of glucose metabolism and chronic morbidity, so called estrogenic diseases [18].

Recent clinical and experimental studies support the concept that estradiol administration is associated with improved insulin sensitivity and appear to be a new therapeutic avenue for patients with type-2 diabetes.

Clinical Data Supporting the Development of Insulin Resistance Induced by Both Estrogen Deficiency and Estrogen Resistance

For many years, estradiol has been considered one of the most important hormones involved in female physiology and reproduction; however, it is now known that its actions are much wider than those previously thought. Estradiol is involved in gene regulation and has important role in several physiologic processes, such as glucose homeostasis in both men and women [1,19].

Rare human cases carrying congenital estrogen deficiency or estrogen resistance have been of fundamental importance in understanding the causal correlation between lack of estrogen signaling and the development of insulin resistance.

Severe mutations of the human aromatase gene (CYP19) were reported in a sister and a brother, both exhibiting extreme estrogen deficiency (20]. The 28-year-old girl presented delayed puberty, progressive signs of virilization and polycystic ovaries with extremely high androgen concentrations in the cystic fluid. Plasma androgen concentrations were highly elevated, whereas plasma estradiol levels were extremely low. Estrogen therapy led to the development of breast, regular menstrual cycles and resolution of the ovarian cysts. This case illuminates that polycystic ovarian syndrome (PCOS), the most frequent hormonal and metabolic disorder in young women may derive from defective estrogen signaling.

The XY male sibling also carrying the CYP19 mutation was examined at 24 years of age [20]. He was 204 cm tall, presenting with macroorchidism. The plasma concentrations of androgens were elevated, while estrogen levels were extremely low. Hyperinsulinemia, increased levels of serum total and low density lipoprotein cholesterol as well as high triglyceride levels were detected suggesting insulin resistance.

Estrogen resistance caused by severe mutation affecting ERs was reported in a 28-year-old man presenting with knock-knees. Examinations revealed his testosterone levels to be normal and, although his estrogen hormone levels were extremely high, he essentially showed no response to estrogen. Signs of serious insulin resistance were apparent such as obesity and premature cardiovascular lesions [21].

In a recently published case an 18-year-old girl presented with delayed puberty alongside the classic symptoms of too low estrogen levels [22].

Subsequent examinations revealed sky-high levels of estrogens in her blood. In laboratory studies, 240 times the normal estrogen level was required to get a response out of the patient's estrogen receptors. Without estrogen reactivity, her insulin levels were also typically increased, and an unusual response to oral glucose test indicated glucose intolerance problems.

Experimental Data Supporting the Upregulating Effect of Estrogen Signaling on Cellular Glucose Uptake

The two ER isoforms, ERα and ERβ, belong to the steroid-thyroid hormone nuclear receptor supergene family [23]. ERs are activated by estradiol and act as transcriptional factors by binding to specific sequences in the promoter region of target genes [24,25]. ERα and ERβ have distinct biologic functions; however, strict crosstalk and interplay have been revealed in their activities.

In HC11 cell line obtained from pregnant mouse mammary glands, selective agonists were used to stimulate ERα and ERβ and it was observed that the agonists for ERα caused cell proliferation, while the agonists for ERβ inhibited the proliferative activity [26].

The development of three knockout mouse lines; ERαKO, ERβKO and ArKO (aromatase knockout) became an important tool for understanding estrogen actions on glucose homeostasis [1]. It was found that mice lacking ERα exhibit insulin resistance, impaired glucose tolerance and adiposity, affecting both males and females. These findings reveal the important role of ERα signaling in the maintenance of glucose homeostasis [27]. Considering the crucial role of ERα signaling in proliferating cellular systems, increased glucose uptake provides essential fuel for energy consuming processes.

In contrast, ERβ seems to have an apparently opposing regulatory action on glucose and insulin metabolism. Ovariectomy of ERαKO mice, which dramatically decreased estrogen synthesis, improved the insulin resistance, suggesting that decreased estrogen signaling may transitorily improve the imbalance between the two ER isoforms [28].

In aromatase knockout (ArKO) mice with inactivation of the enzyme responsible for estrogen synthesis, the importance of estradiol for glucose homeostasis has also been justified [29]. Estrogen deficient ArKO mice present reduced glucose oxidation, increased adiposity and hyperinsulinemia in both males and females [30]. Glucose intolerance and insulin resistance can be reversed by estradiol administration even in male ArKO mice [31].

Molecular Mechanisms of Estrogen Signaling in the Regulation of Cellular Glucose Uptake and Energy Homeostasis

The metabolic state of the body is controlled by a central regulation of the brain through signals arriving from the pancreas, liver, adipose tissue, skeletal muscle, and gut [18]. A wide variety of these signals includes hormones (insulin, leptin, adiponectin, etc.), cytokines (TNF-α, IL-6] and nutrients [glucose, free fatty acids, lipids]. The central nervous system may induce metabolic and behavioral changes by anorexigenic and orexigenic stimuli so as to maintain the serum glucose level and energy homeostasis in the different organs.

The hypothalamic nuclei have a controlling effect on insulin, glucocorticoid and the gonadal hormone functions, which have crucial roles in defining insulin sensitivity and consequently in peripheral carbohydrate and lipid metabolism [17,18,32]. The ratio of male to female sexual hormone levels has particular effect on peripheral fat distribution, which is linked with the modulation of insulin sensitivity. Hyperandrogenism associated with estrogen deficiency or defective estrogen signaling results in insulin resistance and a male-like central, visceral adiposity, while proper estrogen signaling does not affect insulin sensitivity and may be associated with a female-like gluteofemoral deposition of fatty tissue [33].

Estrogen Signaling Defines Insulin Synthesis and Secretion of Pancreatic islets

Pancreatic islets are responsible for insulin synthesis and secretion. Through the insulin signaling pathway, cellular transmembrane insulin receptors (IRs) regulate whole-body glucose homeostasis by transducing extracellular signals to downstream intracellular targets [18].

Estradiol and its receptors are key players in the physiology and insulin production capacity of the β cells of pancreatic islets [15]. Estradiol administration is associated with pancreatic islet hypertrophy and increased insulin release from the β cells in rats. Islet cells isolated from ovariectomized mice respond to glucose with a smaller insulin release than islet cells from intact mice. Estradiol replacement in ovariectomized mice normalizes the insulin response to glucose ingestion [1]. Activation of ER-α promotes β-cell mass proliferation and insulin biosynthesis even in diabetic and obese cases, whereas ER-β activation improves glucose stimulated insulin secretion [16].

In postmenopausal women, low estrogen levels bring about a decrease in insulin sensitivity resulting in an increased inclination to develop obesity and type 2 diabetes. After menopause, reduced insulin secretion is transitorily compensated by the reduced elimination of insulin [34]. During postmenopausal hormone replacement therapy or contraceptive use estradiol improves insulin secretion, sensitivity and elimination.

Estrogen signaling pathways seem to be essential for structural and functional β cell adaptation, especially during periods of high metabolic demand and increased insulin resistance. Recognition of these correlations will lead to novel therapies for β-cell related diseases [17]. Estrogen administration provides a therapeutic possibility of preserving functional β-cell mass in patients with diabetes mellitus.

Estrogen Signaling Regulates Energy Homeostasis in the Liver

Liver function disturbances are in close correlation with insulin resistance, hyperglycemia and dyslipidemia. Estrogen plays a pivotal role in the regulation of glucose homeostasis and insulin sensitivity of mouse liver [35]. ERα is the predominant receptor isoform in hepatocytes and the ERα signal is essential for glucose tolerance and insulin sensitivity in the liver [36].

Glucose homeostasis in the liver is not dependent on intracellular glucose transporters (GLUTs). Insulin modulates hepatic carbohydrate metabolism via direct effects on hepatic enzymatic activities. Glucose uptake is controlled by activation of glycogen synthase and glycogen phosphorylase leading to glucose storage as glycogen in the hepatocytes; whereas insulin may stimulate glycolysis through the activation of several hepatic enzymes [35].

PPT, a selective ERα agonist, improved glucose tolerance and insulin sensitivity in genetically obese mice suggesting that estradiol has antidiabetogenic impact via ERα signaling [37]. In the liver of ERαKO mice, hepatic insulin resistance, increased glucose production and lipid synthesis as well as decreased lipid transport were observed [35]. By contrast ERβ might induce a diabetogenic effect as ERβKO mice with increased body weight exhibited improved hepatic and muscular insulin sensitivity due to reduced accumulation of triglycerides [38].

ERα confers estradiol mediated protection of the liver from inflammatory injuries [39]. Ovariectomized mice were treated by IL-18 to induce hepatic inflammation and estradiol hampered the expression of cytokines in ERβKO but not in ERαKO mice. These data suggest that ERα is the chief regulator of defense against experimental hepatitis.

Estradiol replacement in postmenopausal women increased HDL and decreased LDL, total cholesterol, lipoprotein, fasting insulin and glucose levels, presenting antidiabetogenic and antiatherogenic effects [40]. Nevertheless, estrogen deficiency, such as antiestrogen (tamoxifen) therapy or ovariectomy resulted in atherogenic lipid profile and hepatic steatosis increasing the risk of metabolic syndrome and cardiovascular diseases [41].

Role of Estrogen Signaling in the Energy Homeostasis of Skeletal Muscles

Skeletal muscle mass is responsible for 75% of insulin-mediated glucose uptake in the body [18] consequently, physical activity is in close correlation with insulin sensitivity [42].

Peripheral glucose uptake requires active transport through the double lipid layer of the cell membrane. Insulin receptors have outer α-subunits with binding sites for insulin, whereas the two transmembrane β-subunits are responsible for intracellular signal transduction. Insulin interaction with the external α-subunits induces auto-phosphorylation of β-subunits on multiple tyrosines resulting in an activation of signal transduction [43]. The phosphorylation cascade provokes translocation of glucose transporter (GLUT4) containing cytoplasmic vesicles to the cell membrane. GLUT4 anchored to the cell membrane enables the facilitated diffusion of glucose from the extracellular space into the cell [44]. All these mechanisms, such as insulin supply, insulin signal transduction, GLUT4 expression and intracellular translocation as well as GLUT4-associated cellular glucose uptake are defined by appropriate estrogen signaling [17].

Estradiol stimulates the phosphorylation of Akt, AMPK and the Akt substrate in soleus muscle [45]. Estradiol administration to insulin resistant rats or mice increases the insulin receptor substrate content and the concentration of the phosphorylated form of Akt in muscles, restoring the action of insulin [46,47].

Estrogen receptors are important players in the balance of glucose uptake and energy expenditure [1]. They advantageously modulate insulin stimulated glucose uptake through regulation of the tyrosine phosphorylation of insulin receptor protein [48]. ERs participate in GLUT4 expression and translocation as well. Moreover, estradiol treatment improves glucose homeostasis by way of facilitation GLUT4 incorporation into the cell membrane, resulting in increased GLUT4 content [49]. In ovariectomized rats, the decreased amount of GLUT1 protein in the blood-brain barrier was found to be increased after estradiol substitution [50].

Skeletal muscle expresses both ERs, and in mice ERβ is the predominant isoform. Knowledge on the role of each receptor has been obtained from studies on both receptor knockout mice and use of selective estrogen receptor modulators [18]. Treatment with the ERα selective agonist PPT increased GLUT4 translocation to the cell membrane of L6 myoblasts, while after ERα silencing a decreased translocation was observed [51]. ERα knockout (ERαKO) mice are glucose intolerant and insulin resistant [27] showing that the absence of ERα involves a reduced glucose uptake in muscles [35]. ERβ seems to be a repressor of GLUT4 expression and translocation. In ERβKO mice, both glucose tolerance and insulin release remain normal or better as compared with wild type mice [35,38]. These data support that a steadily balanced activation of both receptor isoforms may ensure the ideal glucose tolerance and energy expenditure.

During estrogen loss in the perimenopausal and postmenopausal periods, muscle strength exhibits a striking decline that can be reversed by hormone replacement therapy (HRT), suggesting that estrogens are important players of muscle physiology [52,53].

Pathologic hyperestrogenism is rare in humans and there are exceedingly controversial findings concerning its correlation with insulin sensitivity. According to certain authors, hyperestrogenism is also related to insulin resistance similarly to estrogen deficiency [54]. In women with irregular menstrual cycles, anovulatory infertility and gestational diabetes, occurrence of hyperestrogenism was presumed to be a contributor to insulin resistance [55,56]. Nevertheless, pathologic insulin resistant states coupled with increased estrogen levels may be regarded as consequences of defective ER signaling and the increased estrogen synthesis is a compensatory process so as to break through the estrogen resistance [57]. When this counteractive estrogen overproduction is not sufficient to maintain cellular estrogen surveillance, insulin resistance may develop, which is attributed to the defect of estrogen signaling rather than hyperestrogenism.

Treatment with pregnancy equivalent estradiol seems to have antidiabetogenic, antiobesity and anticancer effects in animal experiments [58,59]. Moreover, high dose estrogen administration as ovulation provocation and good hormonal equilibrium in multiparous women prove to be metabolically advantageous and exhibit anticancer capacities [9].

Taken together, estrogens have beneficial effects on insulin sensitivity and an estrogen deficient milieu endangers balanced glucose uptake and energy expenditure of skeletal muscles leading to insulin resistance [17].

Role of Estrogen Signaling in the Energy Homeostasis and Deposition of Adipose Tissue

Increased adipose tissue deposition in visceral location has been linked to a self-generating process of insulin resistance. Adipose tissue participates in a variety of metabolic, endocrine and immunologic processes and interacts with central nervous system and peripheral organs by means of adipokine secretion. The size of the fatty tissue compartment clearly reflects the balance between whole-body energy intake and expenditure [60].

In rats, ovariectomy has been found to increase body weight, intra-abdominal fat, fasting glucose, insulin levels and insulin resistance. Estradiol substitution was shown to restore normoglycemia, increase the expression of adiponectin and decrease resistin expression resulting in improvement of insulin sensitivity [61].

In healthy premenopausal women, estradiol counteracts the development of obesity and insulin resistance [62]. Estradiol prevents the accumulation of visceral fat, and decreases the lipogenic activity of lipoprotein lipase in adipose tissue. By contrast, irregular or long menstrual cycles in young women are associated with insulin resistance and predict occurrence of type-2 diabetes by account of a defective estrogen synthesis [63]. After menopause, with decreasing estradiol production and deepening insulin resistance, increased lipid deposition and decreased lipid utilization develop, resulting in visceral fat mass accumulation [64].

The presence of ERα and ERβ isoforms was confirmed in human adipocytes deriving from both subcutaneous and intra-abdominal adipose tissues, with clear predominance of ERα [65]. Although the separated functions of the two ERs in adipose tissue can be studied on disabled ERαKO and ERβKO mice, these results could hardly be extrapolated to human practice. The only clinical case was a 28-year-old man with the genetic defect of ERα who presented with glucose intolerance, hyperinsulinemia and obesity [21]. Hyperestrogenism in this patient seemed to be a contra-regulatory effect. Failure of his ERα signal led to premature coronary artery disease and decreased levels of total, LDL and HDL cholesterol [66].

In male mice, deletion of ERα induced insulin resistance and a progressive increase in adipose tissue with advancing age. In female ERαKO mice, insulin resistance, increased adiposity, higher leptin and cholesterol levels and smaller LDL particles were found to be characteristic [27].

Estradiol substitution in ovariectomized mice kept on high-fat diet, preserved glucose tolerance and insulin sensitivity [47]. Studies on ERα and ERβ knockout mice suggested that ERα is the main regulator of GLUT4 expression in adipose tissue [18] and the two ER isoforms have opposite functions on fat metabolism [28]. In human adipocytes, there is a high correlation between GLUT4 abundance and insulin responsiveness. In PCOS cases with ovarian overproduction of testosterone and defective estrogen synthesis, insulin stimulated glucose uptake was reduced due to decreased amounts of GLUT4 in the adipocyte membrane [67].

Lifelong Changes in Sex Hormone Levels and Their Correlation with Insulin Resistance, Type-2 Diabetes and Obesity in Women

In premenopausal women, the good equilibrium of sexual steroid synthesis defines somatic health and reproductive capacity, whereas good, symptom-free adaptation to the estrogen deficient environment is a prerequisite of postmenopausal health (9,68). During women's lives, the alterations taking place in the sexual hormone equilibrium have strong effect on the insulin sensitivity and associated risks for type-2 diabetes and obesity.

Changes in Sexual Hormone Levels and Insulin Sensitivity in Puberty

In puberty, the extreme somatic growth and explosion-like sexual development are great challenges for the entire metabolic and hormonal systems. During this period there is higher risk for development of insulin resistance, particularly in overweight subjects, induced by either inherited inclination or exogenous noxae. Increased insulin resistance does not return to prepubertal values at the end of puberty, thus representing a high risk for adult metabolic syndrome, type-2 diabetes and further complications [69,70].

In adolescent girls, developing insulin resistance also leads to abnormal ovarian sexual steroidgenesis, resulting in excessive androgen and defective estrogen productions and a higher frequency of menstrual irregularity and anovulatory cycles [71,72,73]. Elevated serum androgen concentrations associated with insulin resistance in adolescents are sustained into adulthood and are reflected by defective fertility patterns at least until 30 years of age [72,73].

Development of pathologic dysmetabolism and hyperandrogenism in the critical period of puberty might be a defining, dangerous factor for later metabolic syndrome, type-2 diabetes and their comorbidities [74].

Correlations between Changes in Estrogen Levels and Insulin Sensitivity in Premenopausal Women

In premenopausal young women, defective estrogen synthesis and decreased estrogen signaling are frequently associated with anovulation and infertility. Long and/or irregular menstrual cycles are the clinical signs of ovarian insufficiency [75,76]. These reproductive dysfunctions are usually related to hyperinsulinism and excessive androgen production [9].

Among premenopausal hormonal disorders with insulin resistance and fertility failure, polycystic ovarian syndrome (PCOS) is the most prevalent entity, most likely caused by a number of different genetic abnormalities [77]. It seems to be a pathologic model of hormonal and metabolic alterations for estrogen deficient postmenopausal status in young women. PCOS may manifest itself via menstrual disorders, anovulatory infertility, hirsutism and obesity or overweight. Nevertheless, polycystic ovaries are common findings in symptom-free cases with apparently normal menstrual cycles as well; only laboratory findings of hyperinsulinemia and hyperandrogenism reveal the early phase of metabolic and hormonal disturbances [78,79].

PCOS is not only an infertility disease but poses a high systemic health risk for affected women as well. Increased prevalence of type-2 diabetes, hypertension and cardiovascular complications were observed in a follow up study of a Dutch population of women with PCOS [63]. Close associations between PCOS and premature coronary and aortic atherosclerosis were revealed in middle-aged women [80,81]. A retrospective Swedish study found a 7.4-fold risk of myocardial infarction among women suffering of PCOS [82].

In young infertile, nulliparous women with or without PCOS, an elevated risk for endometrial cancer was observed [83]. The high prevalence of endometrial cancer is frequently associated with synchronous primary carcinomas of the ovary or breast [83,84]. This female organ triad has the highest demand for estrogen surveillance, attributed to their cyclic proliferative activity, which shows peculiar cancer risk even in a slightly estrogen deficient environment [2,9,85].

Earlier, it was assumed by some authors that elevated estrogen levels unopposed by progestin continuously stimulate estrogen receptors in women with PCOS. This concept seemed to be a plausible explanation for the high risk of endometrial and breast cancers observed in these cases based on the concept of the carcinogenic capacity of estrogen [86]. Recently, insulin resistance and hyperinsulinemia in PCOS patients are regarded as concomitants of high ovarian and adrenal androgen synthesis at the expense of defective estrogen production [87].

In women, hyperprolactinemia is also associated with insulin resistance, obesity, cycle disorders, reproductive dysfunction and hyperandrogenism, however, it should be delineated from PCOS and other disorders related to androgen excess. Glucose intolerance and obesity are characteristic in hyperprolactinemia, suggesting that prolactin or the associated hormonal disturbances might also be modulators of insulin sensitivity and body weight [88,89]. In a population based cohort study the overall cancer risk was found to be elevated in patients with hyperprolactinemia [90].

Oral contraceptive (OC) use replaces the natural menstrual cycle with relatively steady levels and fluctuations of exogenous sex hormones. In PCOS cases, hormone treatment by oral contraceptives reduces the volume of cystic ovaries, decreases testosterone secretion and improves the carbohydrate and lipid metabolism as well [91]. At the same time, administration of the insulin sensitizing metformin in PCOS cases primarily lowers the high insulin level and improves menstrual abnormalities, ovulatory dysfunction and hirsutism [92].

Epidemiologic studies have confirmed that combined oral contraceptive administration provides substantial protection against endometrial and ovarian cancers in endangered anovulatory women [93]. A recent patent disclosed a method for treating hyperandrogenism and associated conditions, including PCOS by an estrogen derivative compound [94]. This therapy seems to have more advantage against the dangerous dysmetabolism of PCOS cases than oral contraceptive administration.

Tamoxifen is a nonsteroidal anti-estrogenic drug used for adjuvant therapy of breast cancer and more recently as a chemopreventive agent for breast cancer and as well as other cancers [95]. Nevertheless, worldwide administration of antiestrogen compounds yielded thorough disappointment [96].

Antiestrogens are cytostatic agents blocking the most important regulatory mechanisms associated with estrogen signaling. They have ambiguous impacts on mammary tumor development, however, the estrogen deprivation induces several life-threatening side-effects and exhibits strong carcinogenic capacity, particularly in the highly estrogen dependent endometrium [97]. Results of case-control studies demonstrated an increased prevalence of fatty liver, intraabdominal fat accumulation and type-2 diabetes in breast cancer cases receiving tamoxifen [95,98,99]. Both artificial blocking of estrogen signaling pathways and estrogen withdrawal seem to confer serious insulin resistance.

Correlations between Estrogen Loss and the Risk of Increasing Insulin Resistance in Postmenopausal Women

Menopause at 50-52 years of age means that there is a sudden loss of ovarian estrogen synthesis together with the decline of the circulating hormone level.

Postmenopausal women never using HRT are obviously insulin resistant and exhibit increasing inclination to the associated comorbidities. With ageing, every year after menopause is associated with continuous estrogen loss and the parallel advance in insulin resistance [100]. For women aged 55-65 years, weight gain and obesity are the major health risks [101]. In postmenopausal women, deepening dysmetabolism, obesity and disturbance of male to female sexual steroid levels are associated with increased prevalence of metabolic syndrome, type-2 diabetes, cardiovascular disease and malignancies.

In HRT user postmenopausal women, the protective effect of estrogen substitution may counteract the developing insulin resistance and the metabolic and hormonal equilibrium of these cases becomes reminiscent to that of young women with preserved circulatory estrogen levels [9]. Estradiol administration increases insulin sensitivity [1], yields favorable changes in plasma lipid levels [102] and its anti-obesity effect reduces fat accumulation, particularly that of visceral adiposity [103,104]. All these impacts justify that

HRT use is beneficially protective against insulin resistance and its comorbidities in postmenopausal women.

Hysterectomy and bilateral oophorectomy mean abrupt, shocking hormone deprivation as compared with natural menopause. Such patients are highly endangered since they are lacking the possibility for gradual adaptation to the estrogen loss by means of a compensatory hormone synthesis of the peripheral tissues [68,85].

Bilateral oophorectomy is used as a risk reduction strategy in BRCA1/2 mutation carriers, although data on long-term side effects are not yet available. In the US population, oophorectomy, particularly at a young age, has been associated with highly increased overall and cardiovascular disease (CVD) mortality rate [105]. In 2011, the WHI Randomized Controlled Trial substantiated that estrogen treatment in women with prior hysterectomy resulted in a significantly lower breast cancer risk as compared with untreated controls [106]. Hysterectomy seems to be a near uniformly high breast cancer risk for women, thus HRT studies on these homogenously selected cases have proved to be methodologically strong yielding unexpectedly correct results [2].

In postmenopausal women, antiestrogen administration is a worldwide practice as either a therapeutic or cancer preventive agent. Both ER-blocker and aromatase inhibitor types of antiestrogens further aggravate the estrogen deficiency and insulin resistance of aged female patients [96]. Transient health maintenance during antiestrogen administration may be attributed to the alarming counteraction against destroyed estrogen signaling by means of extreme peripheral estrogen synthesis and overexpression of ERs. Later on, the exhaustion of forced defensive reactions results in severe toxic effects and tumor development in antiestrogen treated cases. This phase is mistakenly regarded as secondary antiestrogen resistance, whilst essentially it is the total completion of estrogen blockage.

Conclusion

Diverse disorders associated with insulin resistance are usually well treatable by estradiol substitution in both pre- and postmenopausal women as well as animal experiments. Estrogen activated signaling of ER isoforms seems to have balanced interplay in the maintenance of ideal glucose uptake and energy expenditure with continuous adaptation to the momentarily changing intra- and extracellular stimuli. This equilibrium may be shattered in case of a defective estrogen supply or by the derangement of ER signaling pathways.

Considering the advantageous effects of suitable estrogen signaling on insulin secretion, cellular glucose uptake and further metabolic processes, estrogen administration seems to be a new therapeutic possibility to improve insulin sensitivity in patients with metabolic syndrome and diabetes mellitus.

References

[1]   Barros RPA, Machadon UF, Gustafsson JA. Estrogen receptors: new players in diabetes mellitus. *Trends Molecular Med.* 9:425-431, 2006.

[2]   Suba Z. Interplay between insulin resistance and estrogen deficiency as co-activators in carcinogenesis. *Pathol Oncol Res.* 18:123-33, 2012.

[3]   Bloomgarden ZT. The 1st World Congress on the Insulin Resistance Syndrome. *Diabetes Care.* 27(2):602-9, 2004

[4]   Wild S, Roglic G, Green A, Sicree R, King H. Global prevalence of diabetes: estimates for the year 2000 and projections for 2030. *Diabetes Care.* 27(5):1047-53, 2004.

[5]   Reaven GM. Banting lecture 1988: Role of insulin resistance in human disease. *Diabetes.* 37:1595-1607, 1988.

[6]   DeFronzo, R.A., Ferrannini, E. Insulin resistance: a multifaceted syndrome responsible for NIDDM, obesity, hypertension, dyslipidemia and atherosclerotic cardiovascular disease. *Diabetes Care.* 14:173-194, 1991.

[7]   Gupta K, Krishnaswamy G, Karnad A, Peiris A. Insulin: A novel factor in carcinogenesis. *Am J Med Sci.* 323:140-145, 2002.

[8]   Faulds MH, Zhao C, Dahlman-Wright K, Gustaffson J. The diversity of sex steroid action: regulation of metabolism by estrogen signaling. *J Endocrinol.* 212:3-12, 2012.

[9]   Suba Z. Circulatory Estrogen Level Protects Against Breast Cancer in Obese Women. *Recent Pat Anticancer Drug Discov.* 8(2):154-67, 2013.

[10] Reaven GM. Insulin resistance, cardiovascular disease, and the metabolic syndrome: How well do the emperor's clothes fit? *Diabetes Care.* 27:1011-1012, 2004.

[11] Doyle SL, Donohoe CL, Lysaght J, Reynolds JV. Visceral obesity, metabolic syndrome, insulin resistance and cancer. *Proc Nutr Soc.* 71:181-9, 2012.

[12] Pennathur S, Heinecke JW. Mechanisms for oxidative stress in diabetic cardiovascular disease. *Antioxid Redox Signal.* 9:955-69, 2007.

[13] Baynes JW, Thorpe SR. Role of oxidative stress in diabetic complications: a new perspective on an old paradigm. *Diabetes.* 48:1-9 1999.

[14] Altomare E, Vendemiale G, Chicco D, Procacci V, Cirelli F. Increased lipid peroxidation in type 2 poorly controlled diabetic patients. *Diabetes Metab.* 18: 264-71, 1992.

[15] Choi SB, Jang JS, Park S. Estrogen and exercise may enhance beta-cell function and mass via insulin receptor substrate-2 induction in ovariectomized diabetic rats. *Endocrinology.* 146:4786-94, 2005.

[16] Tiano JP, Mauvais-Jarvis F. Importance of oestrogen receptors to preserve functional β-cell mass in diabetes. *Nat Rev Endocrinol.* 8:342-51, 2012.

[17] Suba Z. Low estrogen exposure and/or defective estrogen signaling induces disturbances in glucose uptake and energy expenditure. *J Diabet Metab.* 4:272-81, 2013.

[18] Barros RP, Gustafsson JÅ. Estrogen receptors and the metabolic network. *Cell Metab.* 14:289-99, 2011.

[19] Maggi A. Liganded and unliganded activation of estrogen receptor and hormone replacement therapies. *Biochim Biophys Acta.* 1812(8):1054-60, 2011.

[20] Morishima A, Grumbach MM, Simpson ER, Fisher C, Qin K. Aromatase deficiency in male and female siblings caused by a novel mutation and the physiological role of estrogens. *J Clin Endocrinol Metab.* 80(12):3689-98, 1995.

[21] Smith EP, Boyd J, Frank GR, Takahashi H, Cohen RM, Specker B, Williams TC, Lubahn DB, Korach KS. Estrogen resistance caused by a mutation in the estrogen-receptor gene in a man. *N Engl J Med.* 331:1056–1061, 1994.

[22] Quaynor SD, Stradtman EW, Kim HG, Shen Y, Chorich LP, Schreihofer DA, Layman LC. Delayed Puberty and Estrogen Resistance in a Woman with Estrogen Receptor α Variant. *N Engl J Med.* 369(2):164-171, 2013.

[23] Nilsson S, Mäkelä S, Treuter E, Tujague M, Thomsen J, Andersson G, Enmark E, Pettersson K, Warner M, Gustafsson JA. Mechanisms of estrogen action. *Physiol Rev.* 81(4):1535-65, 2001.

[24] Katzenellenbogen BS. Estrogen receptors: bioactivities and interactions with cell signaling pathways. *Biol Reprod.* 54(2):287-93, 1996.

[25]   Koehler KF, Helguero LA, Haldosén LA, Warner M, Gustafsson JA.
       Reflections on the discovery and significance of estrogen receptor beta.
       Endocr Rev. 26(3):465-78, 2005.

[26]   Helguero LA, Faulds MH, Gustafsson JA, Haldosén LA. Estrogen
       receptors alfa (ERalpha) and beta (ERbeta) differentially regulate
       proliferation and apoptosis of the normal murine mammary epithelial
       cell line HC11. *Oncogene.* 24(44): 6605-16, 2005.

[27]   Heine PA, Taylor JA, Iwamoto GA, Lubahn DB, Cooke PS. Increased
       adipose tissue in male and female estrogen receptor-alpha knockout
       mice. *Proc Natl Acad Sci USA.* 97:12729–12734, 2000.

[28]   Naaz A, Zakroczymski M, Heine P, Taylor J, Saunders P, Lubahn D,
       Cooke PS. Effect of ovariectomy on adipose tissue of mice in the
       absence of estrogen receptor alpha (ERalpha): a potential role for
       estrogen receptor beta (ERbeta). *Horm Metab Res.* 34:758–763, 2002.

[29]   Fisher CR, Graves KH, Parlow AF, Simpson ER. Characterization of
       mice deficient in aromatase (ArKO) because of targeted disruption of the
       cyp19 gene. *Proc Natl Acad Sci USA.* 95:6965-70, 1998.

[30]   Jones ME, Thorburn AW, Britt KL, Hewitt KN, Wreford NG, Proietto J,
       Oz OK, Leury BJ, Robertson KM, Yao S, Simpson ER. Aromatase-
       deficient (ArKO) mice have a phenotype of increased adiposity. *Proc
       Natl Acad Sci USA.* 97:12735-40, 2000.

[31]   Takeda K, Toda K, Saibara T, Nakagawa M, Saika K, Onishi T, Sugiura
       T, Shizuta Y. Progressive development of insulin resistance phenotype
       in male mice with complete aromatase (CYP19) deficiency. *J
       Endocrinol.* 176:237-46, 2003.

[32]   Genabai NK, Briski KP. Adaptation of arcuate insulin receptor, estrogen
       receptor-alpha, estrogen receptor-beta, and type-II glucocorticoid
       receptor gene profiles to chronic intermediate insulin-induced
       hypoglycemia in estrogen-treated ovariectomized female rats. *J Mol
       Neurosci.* 41:304–309, 2010.

[33]   Pallottini V, Bulzomi P, Galluzzo P, Martini C, Marino M. Estrogen
       regulation of adipose tissue functions: involvement of estrogen receptor
       isoforms. *Infect Disord Drug Targets.* 8:52-60, 2008.

[34]   Godsland IF. Oestrogens and insulin secretion. *Diabetologia.* 48:2213–
       2220, 2005.

[35]   Bryzgalova G, Gao H, Ahren B, Zierath JR, Galuska D, Steiler TL, *et al.*
       Evidence that oestrogen receptor-alpha plays an important role in the
       regulation of glucose homeostasis in mice: insulin sensitivity in the liver.
       Diabetologia. 49:588-97, 2006.

[36] Gao H, Fält S, Sandelin A, Gustafsson JA, Dahlman-Wright K. Genome-wide identification of estrogen receptor alpha-binding sites in mouse liver. *Mol Endocrinol.* 22:10–22, 2008.

[37] Lundholm L, Bryzgalova G, Gao H, Portwood N, Fält S, Berndt KD, Dicker A, Galuska D, Zierath JR, Gustafsson JA et al. The estrogen receptor alpha-selective agonist propyl pyrazole triol improves glucose tolerance in ob/ob mice; potential molecular mechanisms. *J Endocrinol.* 199:275–286, 2008.

[38] Foryst-Ludwig A, Clemenz M, Hohmann S, Hartge M, Sprang C, Frost N, Krikov M, Bhanot S, Barros R, Morani A et al. Metabolic actions of estrogen receptor beta (ERbeta) are mediated by a negative cross-talk with PPARgamma. *PLoS Genet.* 4: e1000108, 2008.

[39] Evans MJ, Lai K, Shaw LJ, Harnish DC, Chadwick CC. Estrogen receptor alpha inhibits IL-1beta induction of gene expression in the mouse liver. *Endocrinology.* 143:2559–2570, 2002.

[40] Espeland MA, Marcovina SM, Miller V, Wood PD, Wasilauskas C, Sherwin R, Schrott H, Bush TL. Effect of postmenopausal hormone therapy on lipoprotein(a) concentration. PEPI Investigators. Postmenopausal Estrogen/Progestin Interventions *Circulation.* 97:979–986, 1998.

[41] Redig AJ, Munshi HG. Care of the cancer survivor: metabolic syndrome after hormone-modifying therapy. *Am J Med.* 123:87 e1–e6, 2010.

[42] Spangenburg EE, Wohlers LM, Valencia AP. Metabolic dysfunction under reduced estrogen levels: looking to exercise for prevention. *Exerc Sport Sci Rev.* 40(4):195-203, 2012.

[43] Kasuga M, Hedo JA, Yamada KM, Kahn CR. The structure of insulin receptor and its subunits. Evidence for multiple nonreduced forms and a 210,000 possible proreceptor. *J Biol Chem.* 257:10392-9, 1982.

[44] Zhou L, Chen H, Xu P, Cong LN, Sciacchitano S, Li Y, Graham D, Jacobs AR, Taylor SI, Quon MJ. Action of insulin receptor substrate-3 (IRS-3) and IRS-4 to stimulate translocation of GLUT4 in rat adipose cells. *Mol Endocrinol.* 13:505-14, 1999.

[45] Rogers NH, Witczak CA, Hirshman MF, Goodyear LJ, Greenberg AS. Estradiol stimulates Akt, AMP-activated protein kinase (AMPK) and TBC1D1/4, but not glucose uptake in rat soleus. *Biochem Biophys Res Commun.* 382:646–650, 2009.

[46] Ordóñez P, Moreno M, Alonso A, Llaneza P, Díaz F, González C. 17beta-Estradiol and/or progesterone protect from insulin resistance in

STZ-induced diabetic rats. *J Steroid Biochem Mol Biol.* 111:287–294, 2008.

[47] Riant E, Waget A, Cogo H, Arnal JF, Burcelin R, Gourdy P. Estrogens protect against high-fat diet-induced insulin resistance and glucose intolerance in mice. *Endocrinology.* 150:2109-17, 2009.

[48] Muraki K, Okuya S, Tanizawa Y. Estrogen receptor alpha regulates insulin sensitivity trough IRS-1 thyrosin phosphorylation in mature 3T3-L1 adipocytes. *Endocr J.* 53:841-851, 2006.

[49] Moreno M, Ordoñez P, Alonso A, Díaz F, Tolivia J, González C. Chronic 17beta-estradiol treatment improves skeletal muscle insulin signaling pathway components in insulin resistance associated with aging. *Age (Dordr.)* 32:1–13, 2010.

[50] Shi J, Simpkins JW. 17 beta-Estradiol modulation of glucose transporter 1 expression in blood-brain barrier. *Am J Physiol.* 272:E1016-22, 1997.

[51] Galluzzo P, Rastelli C, Bulzomi P, Acconcia F, Pallottini V, Marino M. 17beta-Estradiol regulates the first steps of skeletal muscle cell differentiation via ER-alpha-mediated signals. *Am J Physiol Cell Physiol.* 297:C1249–C1262, 2009.

[52] Phillips SK, Rook KM, Siddle NC, Bruce SA, Woledge RC. Muscle weakness in women occurs at an earlier age than in men, but strength is preserved by hormone replacement therapy. *Clin Sci.* 84:95–98, 1993.

[53] Greising SM, Baltgalvis KA, Lowe DA, Warren GL. Hormone therapy and skeletal muscle strength: a meta-analysis. *J Gerontol A Biol Sci Med Sci.* 64:1071–1081, 2009.

[54] Livingstone C, Collison M. Sex steroids and insulin resistance. *Clin Sci.* 102:151–166, 2002.

[55] Garvey TL, Maianu JH, Zhu W, Hancock JA. Golichowski AM. Multiple defects in the adipocyte glucose transport system cause cellular insulin resistance in gestational diabetes. Heterogeneity in the number and a novel abnormality in subcellular localization of GLUT4 glucose transporters. *Diabetes.* 42:1773–1785, 1993.

[56] Okuno S, Akazawa S,Yasuhi I, Kawasaki E, Matsumoto K, Yamasaki H, Matsuo H, Yamaguchi Y,Nagataki S. Decreased expression of the GLUT4 glucose transporter protein in adipose tissue during pregnancy. *Horm Metab Res.* 27:231–234, 1995.

[57] Suba Z. Diverse pathomechanisms leading to the breakdown of cellular estrogen surveillance and breast cancer development: new therapeutic strategies. *Drug Des Devel Ther.* 8:1381-90, 2014.

[58] Nkhata KJ, Ray A, Dogan S, Grande JP, Cleary MP. Mammary tumor development from T47-D human breast cancer cells in obese ovariectomized mice with and without estradiol supplements. *Breast Cancer Res Treat.* 114:71-83, 2009.

[59] Hong J, Holcomb VB, Kushiro K, Núñez NP. Estrogen inhibits the effects of obesity and alcohol on mammary tumors and fatty liver. *Int J Oncol.* 39:1443-53, 2011.

[60] Frayn KN, Karpe F, Fielding BA, Macdonald IA, Coppack SW. Integrative physiology of human adipose tissue. *Int J Obes Relat Metab Disord.* 27:875–888, 2003.

[61] Kim JY, Jo KJ, Kim OS, Kim BJ, Kang DW, Lee KH, H.W. Baik, M.S. Han, S.K. Lee. Parenteral 17beta-estradiol decreases fasting blood glucose levels in non-obese mice with short-term ovariectomy. *Life Sci.* 87:358–366, 2010.

[62] Clegg DJ, Brown LM, Woods SC, Benoit SC. Gonadal hormones determine sensitivity to central leptin and insulin. *Diabetes.* 55:978-87, 2006.

[63] Elting MW, Korsen TJ, Bezemer PD, Schoemaker J. Prevalence of diabetes mellitus, hypertension and cardiac complaints in a follow-up study of a Dutch PCOS population. *Hum Reprod.* 16:556-60, 2001.

[64] Wohlers LM, Spangenburg EE. 17beta-estradiol supplementation attenuates ovariectomy-induced increases in ATGL signaling and reduced perilipin expression in visceral adipose tissue. *J Cell Biochem.* 110:420–427, 2010.

[65] Dieudonné MN, Leneveu MC, Giudicelli Y, Pecquery R. Evidence for functional estrogen receptors alpha and beta in human adipose cells: regional specificities and regulation by estrogens. *Am J Physiol Cell Physiol.* 286:C655-61, 2004.

[66] Sudhir K, Chou TM, Chatterjee K, Smith EP, Williams TC, Kane JP, Malloy MJ, Korach KS, Rubanyi GM. Premature coronary artery disease associated with a disruptive mutation in the estrogen receptor gene in a man. *Circulation.* 96:3774–3777, 1997.

[67] Rosenbaum D, Haber RS, Dunaif A. Insulin resistance in polycystic ovary syndrome: decreased expression of GLUT-4 glucose transporters in adipocytes. *Am J Physiol.* 264:E197-202, 1993.

[68] Suba Z. Common soil of smoking-associated and hormone-related cancers: estrogen deficiency. *Oncol Rev.* 4:73-87, 2010.

[69] Theintz G. From obesity to type-2 diabetes in children and adolescents. *Rev Med Suisse.* 1:477-80, 2005.

[70] Vanhala MJ, Vanhala PT, Keinänen-Kiukaanniemi SM, Kumpusalo EA, Takala JK. Relative weight gain and obesity as a child predict metabolic syndrome as an adult. *Int J Obes Relat Metab Disord.* 23:656-9, 1999.

[71] Stoll BA. Teenage obesity in relation to breast cancer risk. *Int J Obes Relat Metab Disord.* 22:1035-40, 1998.

[72] Apter D, Vihko R. Endocrine determinants of fertility: serum androgen concentrations during follow-up of adolescents into the third decade of life. *J Clin Endocrinol Metab.* 71:970-4, 1990.

[73] Baer HJ, Colditz GA, Willett WC, Dorgan JF. Adiposity and sex hormones in girls. *Cancer Epidemiol Biomarkers Prev.* 16:1880-8, 2007.

[74] Lewy VD, Danadian K, Witchel SF, Arslanian S, : Early metabolic abnormalities in adolescent girls with polycystic ovarian syndrome. *J Pediatrics.* 138:38-44, 2001.

[75] Zain MM, Norman RJ. Impact of obesity on female fertility and fertility treatment. *Women's Health (Lond Engl).* 4:183-94, 2008.

[76] Rose DP, Vona-Davis L. Interaction between menopausal status and obesity in affecting breast cancer risk. *Maturitas* 66:33-8, 2010.

[77] Bloomgarden ZT. Second World Congress on the Insulin Resistance Syndrome: Mediators, pediatric insulin resistance, the polycystic ovary syndrome, and malignancy. *Diab Care.* 28:1821-1830, 2005.

[78] Polson DW, Wadsworth J, Adams J et al. Polycystic ovaries: a common finding in normal women. *Lancet.* 1:870-872, 1988.

[79] Carmina E, Lobo RA. Polycystic ovaries in hirsute women with normal menses. *Am J Med.* 111:602-606, 2001.

[80] Talbott E, Guzick D, Clerici A, et al. Coronary heart disease risk factors in women with polycystic ovary syndrome. *Arteroscler Thromb Vasc Biol.* 15:821-826, 1995.

[81] Talbott EO, Zborowski JV, Rager JR, Boudreaux MY, Edmundowicz DA, Guzick DS. Evidence for an association between metabolic cardiovascular syndrome and coronary and aortic calcification among women with polycystic ovary syndrome. *J Clin Endocrinol Metab.* 89:5454-5461, 2004.

[82] Dahlgren E, Johansson S, Lindstedt G, et al. Women with polycystic ovary syndrome wedge resected in 1956 to 1975: a long-term follow-up focusing on natural history and circulating hormones. *Fertil Steril.* 57:505-513, 1992.

[83] Soliman PT, Oh JC, Schmeler KM, Sun CC, Slomovitz BM, Gershenson DM, *et al.* Risk factors for young premenopausal women with endometrial cancer. *Obstet Gynecol.* 10:575-80, 2005.

[84] Uccella S, Cha SS, Melton LJ 3rd, Bergstralh EJ, Boardman LA, Keeney GL, *et al.* Risk factors for developing multiple malignancies in patients with endometrial cancer. *Int J Gynecol Cancer.* 21:896-901, 2011.

[85] Suba Zs. Discovery of estrogen deficiency as common cancer risk factor for highly and moderately estrogen dependent organs. In: Ed. Suba Zs. *Estrogen prevention for breast cancer.* Chapter 1. Nova Science Publishers Inc. New York. 2013.

[86] Gadducci A, Gargini A, Palla E, Fanucchi A, Genazzani AR. Polycystic ovary syndrome and gynecological cancers: is there a link? *Gynecol Endocrinol.* 20:200-208, 2005.

[87] Christakou CD, Diamanti-Kandarakis E. Role of androgen excess on metabolic aberrations and cardiovascular risk in women with polycystic ovary syndrome. *Womens Health (Lond Engl).* 4:583-94, 2008.

[88] Tuzcu A, Yalaki S, Arikan S, Gokalp D, Bahcec M, Tuzcu S. Evaluation of insulin sensitivity in hyperprolactinemic subjects by euglycemic hyperinsulinemic clamp technique. *Pituitary.* 12:330-334, 2009.

[89] Shibli-Rahhal A, Schlechte J. The effects of hyperprolactinemia on bone and fat. *Pituitary.* 12:96-104, 2009.

[90] Berinder K, Akre O, Granath F, Hulting AL. Cancer risk in hyperprolactinemia patients: a population-based cohort study. *Eur J Endocrinol.* 165:209-15, 2011.

[91] ESHRE Capri Workshop Group. Ovarian and endometrial function during hormonal contraception. *Hum Reprod.* 16:1527-35, 2001.

[92] Nestler JE. Obesity, insulin, sex steroids and ovulation. *Int J Obes Relat Metab Disord.* 24 Suppl 2: S71-3, 2000.

[93] Deligeoroglou E, Michailidis E, Creatsas G. Oral contraceptives and reproductive system cancer. *Ann NY Acad Sci.* 997:199-208, 2003.

[94] Tejura, B. Methods of treating hyperandrogenism and conditions associated therewith by administering a fatty acid ester of an estrogen or an estrogen derivative. *US20100286105* (2010).

[95] Nguyen MC, Stewart RB, Banerji MA, Gordon DH, Kral JG. Relationships between tamoxifen use, liver fat and body fat distribution in women with breast cancer. *Int J Obes Relat Metab Disord.* 25:296-8, 2001.

[96] Suba Z. Antiestrogen or estrogen as anticancer drug. In: Hoffmann AB. Ed. *Sex hormones: development, regulation and disorders.* Chapter 4. Pp. 75-94. New York, Nova Science Publishers Inc., 2011.

[97] Suba Z. Failures and controversies of the antiestrogen treatment of breast cancer. In: Suba Z. Ed. *Estrogen prevention for breast cancer.* Chapter 6. Nova Science Publishers Inc. New York, 2013.

[98] Saphner T, Triest-Robertson S, Li H, Holzman P. The association of nonalcoholic steatohepatitis and tamoxifen in patients with breast cancer. *Cancer.* 115:3189-95, 2009.

[99] Lipscombe LL, Fischer HD, Yun L, Gruneir A, Austin P, Paszat L, Anderson GM, Rochon PA. Association between tamoxifen treatment and diabetes: a population-based study. *Cancer.* 118:2615-22, 2012.

[100] Schneider JG, Tompkins C, Blumenthal RS, Mora S. The metabolic syndrome in women. *Cardiol Rev.* 14:286-291, 2006.

[101] Davis SR, Castelo-Branco C, Chedraui P, Lumsden MA, Nappi RE, Shah D, Villaseca P; Writing Group of the International Menopause Society for World Menopause Day 2012. Understanding weight gain at menopause. *Climacteric.* 15:419-29, 2012.

[102] Walsh BW, Schiff I, Rosner B, Greenberg L, Ravnikar V, Sacks FM. Effects of postmenopausal estrogen replacement on the concentrations and metabolism of plasma lipoproteins. *N Engl J Med.* 325:1196-204, 1991.

[103] Gunter MJ, Hoover DR, Yu H, Wassertheil-Smoller S, Rohan TE, Manson JE, *et al.* Insulin, insulin-like growth factor and risk of breast cancer in postmenopausal women. *J Natl Cancer Inst.* 101:48-60, 2009.

[104] Tchernof A, Calles-Escandon J, Sites CK, Poehlman ET. Menopause, central body fatness and insulin resistance: effects of hormone-replacement therapy. *Coron Artery Dis.* 9:503-11, 1998.

[105] McCarthy AM, Menke A, Ouyang P, Visvanathan K. Bilateral oophorectomy, body mass index, and mortality in U.S. women aged 40 years and older. *Cancer Prev Res (Phila).* 5:847-54, 2012.

[106] LaCroix AZ, Chlebowski RT, Manson JE, Aragaki AK, Johnson KC, Martin L, *et al.* Health outcomes after stopping conjugated equine estrogens among postmenopausal women with prior hysterectomy. A randomized controlled trial. *JAMA* 305:1305-14, 2011.

In: Impaired Glucose Tolerance ...
Editor: Sandra Wagner

ISBN: 978-1-63483-085-0
© 2015 Nova Science Publishers, Inc.

Chapter 3

Nutritional Management during Perioperative Period: Focusing on Glucose Metabolism and Insulin Sensitivity

Takeshi Yokoyama, DDS, PhD[*]
and Kunio Suwa, MD, PhD[#]

[1] Professor, Department of Dental Anesthesiology,
Faculty of Dental Science, Kyushu University
Higashi-ku, Fukuoka, Japan
[2]Professor, Teikyo Junior College
Shibuya-ku, Tokyo, Japan

Abstract

Surgery is invasive, and injures the patient's physiology. Insulin resistance after surgery increases as the surgical procedure become extensive. Noxious stimuli activate sympathetic nerve system, causing inflammation. It also decreases the insulin sensitivity. Furthermore, hemodynamic changes caused by anesthesia, by bleeding from surgical procedure, and/or by hypothermia result in a stress.

[*] Email: yokoyama@dent.kyushu-u.ac.jp.
[#] Email: kunio.suwa@nifty.com.

After surgery, wound repair is required and the increase in catabolism must be kept minimal. In this view of point, appropriate nutritional management during perioperative period helps prevent catabolism. Blood glucose concentration was recognized recently as an important factor influencing to the outcome. Intensive insulin therapy, however, is not agreed is not upon universally. Shortage of glucose induces glyconeogenesis from amino acids and /or lipids, further causing extensive catabolism. For reducing this, glucose administration is important as well as a good static blood glucose level.

Protocols like ERAS (Enhanced Recovery After Surgery) were being proposed for quick recovery after surgery. This recommends drinking 400 mL of clear water containing carbohydrate 2 hours before anesthesia, but it does not include glucose administration during surgery. For prolonged surgery, patients obviously need good nutritional support. A small dose of glucose during surgery effectively suppresses ketogenesis, and attenuates postoperative insulin resistance.

In this chapter, we intend to describe the amount of carbohydrate required for the day of surgery, and the way to give carbohydrate. We propose a method of evaluating insulin sensitivity after surgery.

Introduction

It is the intent of this chapter to summarize the problems and how to dissolve them. There are three major problems for nutritional management during perioperative period. The first is hyperglycemia, caused by suppression of the immune function [1, 2].

It results in reperfusion injury in the tissues, leading to the poor outcome of surgery [3-8]. The second is fasting. Patients are not allowed to take any food for 6 hours before general anesthesia in order to avoid vomiting during anesthetic induction. Recently, they may be permitted to drink some clear water until 2 hours before the induction of anesthesia, but nutrients and calories are still restricted. The third is a decrease in insulin sensitivity after surgery [9].

This is called "surgical diabetes". Surgical invasion and inadequate nutritional management is the cause of this insulin resistance, leading to the postoperative complications [10]. In addition to these three major problems, overfeeding is recently suggested as a factor affecting the outcome after surgery.

A good nutritional plan before surgery is required for patients with serious systemic illness and/or undergoing surgery with severe invasion, and metabolic condition should be evaluated during perioperative period.

Anesthetic Management without Glucose

In surgery in general and especially in neurosurgery, hyperglycemia has been considered to result in poor outcome. It suppresses neutrophil activity, and causes reperfusion injury of the tissues of major organs [3-8]. High concentration of blood glucose is known to affects the neurologic outcome significantly. Control of blood glucose improves outcome in patients with subarachnoid hemorrhage. Van den Berghe et al. succeeded in reducing morbidity and mortality of critically ill patients in surgical intensive care unit by intensive insulin therapy to maintain blood glucose not more than 110 mg/dL [11]. We must make good effort to keep blood glucose concentration normal.

Hyperglycemia is often caused by infusion with high concentration of glucose of 2.5% to 10% during surgery [12-15]. Furthermore, it had been proposed that glucose administration might not always be necessary during surgery [16-18]. There are several studies suggesting that glucose administration during surgery could be harmful [6, 19, 20]. Until recently, therefore, glucose was avoided during surgery to avoid hyperglycemia, except cases of infants or patients with severe diabetes.

Glucose, in fact, is necessary for biological activity even under general anesthesia, especially in the central nervous system, in red blood cells and in kidney medulla. For 70 kg of men, brain consumes around 120 g of glucose a day. 200 g of glucose is required without muscle exercise. Glucose is stored as glycogen in the body, but the total amount of glycogen is not sufficient for basal metabolism even for one day. Shortage of glucose induces gluconeogenesis mainly in the liver [21]. Gluconeogenesis uses amino acids and/or glycerol as raw materials. There are various glucogenic amino acids, of which, after deamination, carbon structure is utilized for around 90% of gluconeogenesis via pyruvate or oxaloacetate. Glycelol is utilized as the materials for the remaining 10% of gluconeogenesis. Fatty acids are oxidated in mitochondria of the liver. Ketonemia is caused by acceleration of ketogenesis in the liver. In other words, ketonemia indicates shortage of glucose [22]. Too much glucose is utilized for steatgenesis. Therefore, appropriate administration is important especially during perioperative period.

Both hyperglycemia and hypoglycemia should be avoided during perioperative period. It is wrong to disregard nutritional condition. Contrary to the report by van den Berge, NICE SUGAR study investigators reported that the intensive glucose control increased mortality among adults in the ICU [23]. Controversy focusing only on blood glucose concentration is apparently meaningless.

We reported that anesthetic management without glucose increases serum ketone bodies [24]. In patients undergoing orthopedic surgery, ketonemia, observed in a few hours from the start of surgery, was effectively avoided by 1.0% glucose infusion. Yamasaki et al. also reported similar results in patients undergoing head and neck surgery [25]. In addition, Mikura et al reported that infusion without glucose induced muscle protein breakdown in rat model [26].

Evaluation of Insulin Resistance

The third problem is a decrease in insulin sensitivity after surgery. The physiological condition is similar to diabetes, and is called insulin resistance. The pancreas produces insulin, but the tissue cells cannot use it effectively.

There are 2 major methods to evaluate insulin resistance. The standard method for the evaluation of insulin resistance is the normoglycemic hyperinsulinemic clamp technique (glucose clamp) [27]. Insulin is administered continuously at the rate of 80-100 mU/m^2/min to keep hyperinsulinemic condition [28, 29]. Glucose is administered to maintain blood glucose concentration at 90-100mg/dL. The glucose infusion rate (GIR) is used as the indicator of insulin resistance. However, this glucose clamp is complex, and impractical for large human studies.

As a dose of insulin used for glucose clamp is quite large, it is not easy to keep blood glucose appropriate level. We should pay strict attention for avoiding hypoglycemia. The artificial pancreas, STG-22 ^{TM} (Nikkiso Co Ltd.) made glucose clamp semi-automatic. This instrument equips continuous monitor of blood glucose and closed loop system for blood glucose control [30]. By sampling blood continuously (less than 2ml/hr) it monitors blood glucose accurately [31, 32]. Glucose clamp using the STG-22^{TM} was safe and reliable, since GIR was evaluated during steady-state period under constant insulin infusion. STG-55^{TM} (Nikkiso Co Ltd.), next-generation model of STG-22 ^{TM}, became available recently. This device is easier to use than STG-22 ^{TM}.

Another method is homeostasis model assessment insulin resistance (HOMA-IR), which is frequently employed in daily practice as a simple index of insulin resistance.

HOMA-IR = Fasting Insulin (micro-U/mL) x Fasting Blood Sugar (mg/dL) /405.

Two factors multiplying into HOMA-IR are counteracting with each other, and HOMA-IR may be expected to reach a constant value. It is simple and convenient, adaptable for clinical practice and good for evaluation of insulin sensitivity regularly in outpatients. The value of HOMA-IR correlates with GIR of glucose clamp. However, it is inappropriate for perioperative insulin resistance. HOMA-IR requires stable patients condition, since HOMA-IR is determined only by the relation between fasting insulin and fasting blood glucose [33]. However, surgical invasion may increase secretion of stress hormones, and confuse insulin and glucose relation. Therefore, HOMA-IR cannot detect the insulin resistance after surgery. HOMA-IR should not be used to evaluate insulin resistance during perioperative period [34].

In conclusion, glucose clamp is still gold standard for evaluation of perioperative insulin resistance, and glucose clamp using STG-55 is to be recommended.

Artificial Pancreas, STG-22 and STG-55

Artificial pancreas is a feed back control instrument, which consists of 3 units; measurement unit (sensor), control unit (computer) and infusion unit (pumps). Blood glucose concentration is continuously monitored by sampling blood from peripheral vein at less than 2 ml/hr through dual lumen catheter at measurement unit, to which a glucose sensor is incorporated. The information of blood glucose transmitted to the control unit, containing original algorithm [35]. It calculates an appropriate infusion speed of insulin and/or of glucose so as to achieve the setting condition. Yamashita et al. reported the reliability of the glucose measurement during and after surgery [31, 32].

Artificial pancreases, STG-22 and STG-55 [photo 1], are proved to be useful for maintaining optimal blood glucose levels with no hypo- or hyper-glycemia in patients admitted to the intensive care unit. The use of this instrument also helps decrease variability in blood glucose concentration [36, 37]. In addition, these instruments made the intensive insulin therapy easier [38].

These instruments are useful not only for controlling blood glucose, but also for performing glucose clamp examination. Here, the glucose clamp technique is semi-automated, and both hyper- and hypo-glycemia can be avoided effectively. Insulin is administered continuously at the rate of 1.25 mU/kg/min to keep hyperinsulinemic condition [39]. Glucose is administered to maintain blood glucose concentration at 90 mg/dL. The GIR is evaluated as insulin resistance [photo 2]. Nikkiso Co. has developed these instruments, and is advocated it as a bedside-type artificial endocrine pancreas, STG-22, since 1987. STG-55 became available since 2014.

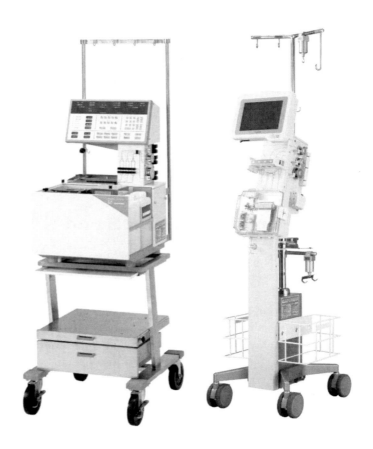

Photo 1. Artificial pancreas STG-22 (left) and STG-55 (right).

Insulin Resistance during Perioperative Period

Insulin is an anabolic hormone. Brandi reported that 8 times more insulin is needed after surgery than before surgery to maintain normal blood sugar level in 1990 [9]. The post-operative insulin resistance increases according to the magnitude of surgical invasion [40]. Thorell compared an increase in insulin resistance between open cholecystectomy and surgical repair of inguinal hernia.

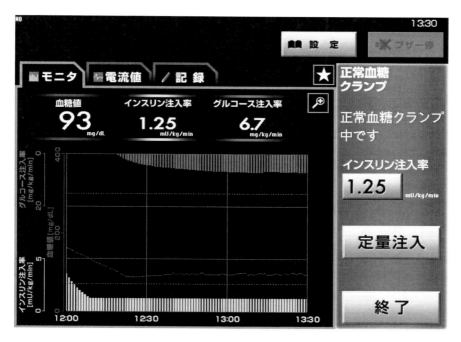

Photo 2. Display screen of STG-55, Red line indicates blood glucose concentration, yellow bar indicates insulin infusion rate and blue bar indicates glucose infusion rate (GIR).

The mechanism of insulin resistance is still unclear. Surgical stress may be inhibiting phosphorylation of insulin receptor, and subsequently suppress transfer of glucose transporter 4 (GLUT4) from cytoplasm to cell membrane. The increase in insulin resistance may lead to the risk of complications after surgery 7. During perioperative period, appropriate nutritional management and the control of insulin resistance are mandatory.

Some methods have been suggested to control insulin resistance after surgery. Preoperative supplementation of carbohydrates attenuates the postoperative insulin resistance [41, 42]. Recently, Yatabe et al. reported that oral intake of carbohydrate in the morning increases insulin sensitivity at 2 hours later [43]. It may depend on the dose of carbohydrate [44]. We reported that low-dose glucose infusion during surgery suppress ketogenesis and attenuates insulin resistance significantly after surgery without causing hyperglycemia [45]. Glucose clamp was performed twice on the day before surgery and on the next day after. The changes of GIR were evaluated as postoperative insulin resistance. By using STG-22 ^{TM} or STG-55 ^{TM}, glucose concentrations were maintained within 90-100mg/dL. GIR decreased by 43.3% in the patients received low-dose glucose (mean administration speed: 0.15g/kg/hr) after overnight fasting, while it decreased by 57.7% in the control patients.

The combination of preoperative carbohydrate and glucose administration during surgery may have synergistic effects on postoperative insulin resistance.

Energy Expenditure during Perioperative Period

Basal energy expenditure (BEE) indicates the energy required for fundamental metabolic functions, such as breathing, circulation and normal turnover of body components for one day [46]. Resting energy expenditure (REE) represents the amount of calories required for one day by the body under non-active condition, which corresponds to around 120% of BEE. Yatabe et al. reported that the REE measured by an indirect calorimeter after minimally invasive esophagectomy at early postoperative stage under sedation was significantly lower than the REE [47]. The average value was less than 1000 kcal. Our data during anesthesia were also from 800 to 1000 kcal/day (data not shown).

Gamble described that at least 100 g of glucose are necessary to avoid severe muscle protein breakdown [48]. At less than 100 g of glucose, catabolism of proteins was suppressed according to the dose of glucose. These data suggested that the amount of calories should be from 400 to 1000 kcal/day under anesthesia or sedated condition. In other words, glucose from 100 to 250 g/day is required. Shortage of calories (underfeeding) may increase the risk of bloodstream infections [49].

Total metabolic calories = external calories + internal calories.

Glyconeogenesis increases to 3.06 mg/kg/min or around 4.4 g/kg/day in the case of septicemic patients. High-dose of glucose administration does not suppress this excessive glyconeogenesis. On the contrary, it may cause marked hyperglycemia [50]. It may be difficult to control the excessive endogenous production of glucose even by insulin [51]. If hyperglycemia were to be avoided, excessive exogenous calories (overfeeding) only increase the risk of infection and deteriorate the outcome [52, 53].

Surgical invasion also induces stress hormone release, accelerates catabolism, and produces endogenous calorie expenditure. External calories should be restricted, if surgical stress is not controlled. Recently, however, surgical stress was shown to be suppressed appropriately by epidural analgesia, by peripheral nerve blocks and/or by strong short-acting opioid analgesics. Then, we may set the goal of glucose dose between 150 and 200g/day for patients undergoing elective surgery according body size and age on the operation day. In addition, body temperature is an important factor. It influences on the metabolism and immuno-activity.

Preoperative Oral Carbohydrate Intake

Overnight fasting had been routine to empty the stomach for avoiding vomiting during induction of anesthesia. Yet, glucose is needed for activity of the brain, of kidney medulla and of red blood cells. However, storage of glucose is restricted, and carbohydrate rich beverage in the morning of surgery is required to maintain insulin sensitivity [54].

Recently the concept of enhanced recovery after surgery spread widely. Clear beverage is permitted until 2 hours before anesthesia. Preoperative oral carbohydrate is important, since much dose of glucose infusion during and after surgery may cause hyperglycemia.

It is reasonable to request empty stomach at the induction of anesthesia. The rate of gastric emptying of liquids should be taken into consideration for preoperative oral carbohydrate intake. However, beverage containing milk protein, some amino acids and/or fibers are likely to prolong them to be discharged from the stomach [55]. For carbohydrate solution, the rate of gastric emptying depends on calories [56, 57]. The lowest safety limit is 100 kcal/hr, and the beverage containing 200 kcal (50 g) of carbohydrate is acceptable for preoperative intake. Then glucose concentration of PreOP solution is 12.5%, and 400 mL of this solution contains 50 g of carbohydrate.

Surgical invasion induces stress hormones, and decrease insulin sensitivity, and inhibits exogenous glucose consumption. While endogenous energy increases, exogenous energy should be restricted to avoid overfeeding in high-risk surgery. Glucose administration during and after surgery should be restricted. Therefore, preoperative carbohydrates intake is important. Oral intake of 50 g of carbohydrate should be an objective for perioperative nutritional management.

Oral Rehydration Solution

In Japan, an oral rehydration solution, OS-1, is commonly as preoperative beverage, which is a strange custom. Oral rehydration solution is defined as a solution containing 40-60 mEq/L of Na^+ and glucose equal to twice high molecular concentration to Na^+ concentration. It is useful for rehydrating the fluid loss to diarrhea or high fever.

OS-1 contains carbohydrates 25 g/L. To take 50 g of carbohydrates, therefore, patients need to take 2 litter of OS-1. Many anesthesiologists believe that OS-1 is useful and safe as preoperative beverage for its fast gastric emptying rate. However, there is no evidence of validity except for thirst. On the contrary, too much of this fluid might be harmful considering recent infusion strategy [58].

Preoperative beverage should be taken easily by patients, as well as containing 50 g of carbohydrate. Oral rehydration solution mentioned above does not match the condition, and should not be recommended for preoperative administration.

Glucose Infusion during Surgery

ESPEN guidelines on parenteral nutrition recommended about 2g/kg/day of glucose as the minimal amount of carbohydrate in intensive care [59]. This administration speed corresponds to around 0.08 g/kg/hr. Glucose administration at 0.08 g/kg/hr suppresses increase in ketone bodies after surgery in spite of postoperative insulin resistance [45]. However, glucose administration during surgery at this speed is not sufficient to suppress the increase in ketone bodies, while mean administration speed at 0.15 g/kg/hr, twice that of above mentioned, suppressed ketogenesis in elective orthopedic surgery [24].

Analgesia is an important factor of anesthesia. Sufficient analgesia could maintain stress hormones at low level. Remifentanil, a short-acting opioid, attenuates hyperglycaemic response [60]. In addition, high-dose remifentanil suppressed both sympathetic responses and the hypothalamus-pituitary-adrenal axis [61]. Postoperative analgesia also important. Good analgesics are obtainable, and patient control analgesia may be a useful approach.

In the cases with sufficient control of surgical invasion, glucose should be administered at 0.1-0.2 g/kg/hr during surgery and at 0.08-0.1 g/kg/hr after surgery. With insufficient analgesia, however, hyperglycemia may be developed with no glucose administration. Some cases still have problems. Insulin sensitivity may have been decreased before surgery, for example, in emergency surgery for patients with severe inflammation and/or severe trauma. Stress control might be difficult in some cardiac surgery using a heart-lung machine.

Nutritional Plan for Patients with Diabetes

Nutritional plan is important for diabetic patients as both hyper- or hypo-glycemia occurs frequently. Any abnormalities of glucose lead to poor outcome. Both hyper- and hypo-glycemia and increased glycemic variability should be avoided. Patients with diabetes may be controlled at higher glucose target ranges than those without diabetes [62].

Objective of glucose dose might not need to change, but glucose concentration should be maintained at higher range according to the usual status for each patient. Insulin might be necessary for some patients, and it should be administered to maintain the target range of glucose concentration.

Conclusion: Seamless Nutritional Management

There are many factors to be considered for attenuating postoperative insulin resistance and for improving the surgical outcome. Appropriate nutritional management, as well as good anesthetic management, is mandatory. Preoperative carbohydrate and glucose infusion during surgery is essential for maintaining insulin sensitivity. Total dose of glucose on the day of surgery is important.

Seamless nutritional management should be planned for patients undergoing operation.

In elective surgery without extremely severe invasion like heart-lung machine, objective of preoperative carbohydrate is 50 g (200 kcal). Anesthesia should achieve good analgesia, and Ringer solution containing 1.0-2.0% of glucose should be infused at the rate of 0.1-0.2 g/kg/hr of glucose. After surgery, 5.0% of glucose solution should be used, and infusion rate should be decreased down to 0.08-0.1 g/kg/hr. According to age and weight, objective of total glucose dose should be set at 150-200g on the operation day. In the cases of severe surgical procedure such as cardiac surgery and/or in the cases with severe inflammation, administration dose of glucose might be restricted to avoid overfeeding since endogenous glucose may increase spontaneously.

References

[1]   J. D. Bagdade, R.K. Root, R.J. *Bulger, Diabetes*. 23, 9 (1974).
[2]   W. Marhoffer, M. Stein, E. Maeser, K. Federlin, *Diabetes Care*. 15, 256 (1992).
[3]   W. A. Pulsinelli, D.E. Levy, B. Sigsbee, P. Scherer, F. Plum, *Am. J. Med.* 74:540 (1983).
[4]   J. E. Fleischer, K. Nakakimura, J.C. Drummond, M.R. Grafe, H.M. Shapiro, *J. Neurosurg. Anesthesiol.* 1, 123 (1989).
[5]   L. Berger, A.M. Hakim, *Stroke,* 17, 865 (1986).
[6]   K. Nakakimura, J.E. Fleischer, J.C. Drummond, M.S. Scheller, M.H. Zornow, M.R. Grafe, H.M. Shapiro, *Anesthesiology,* 72:1005 (1990)
[7]   M.R. Hemmila, G.B. Zelenock, L.G. D'Alecy, *J. Vasc. Surg.* 17, 661 (1993).
[8]   M. Moursi, C. L. Rising, G.B. Zelenock, L. G. D'Alecy, *Arch. Surg.* 122, 790 (1987).
[9]   L. S. Brandi, M, Frediani, M. Oleggini, F. Mosca, M. Cerri, C. Boni, N. Pecori, G. Buzzigoli, E. Ferrannini, *Clin. Sci* (Lond), 79, 443 (1990)
[10] H. Sato, G. Carvalho, T. Sato, R. Lattermann, T. Matsukawa, T. Schricker, *J. Clin. Endocrinol. Metab.* 95, 4338- (2010).

[11] G. van den Berghe, P. Wouters, F. Weekers, C. Verwaest, F. Bruyninckx, M. Schetz, D. Vlasselaers, P. Ferdinande, P. Lauwers, R. Bouillon, *N. Engl. J. Med.* 345, 1359 (2001).

[12] F. E. Sieber, D.S. Smith, J. Kupferberg, L. Crosby, B. Uzzell, G. Buzby, K. March, L. Nann, *Anesthesiology*, 64, 453 (1986).

[13] E.S. Walsh, C. Traynor, J.L. Paterson, G.M. Hall, *Br. J. Anesth.* 55, 135 (1983).

[14] R. Lattermann, F. Carli, L. Wykes, T. Schricker, *Anesth. Analg.* 96, 555 (2003).

[15] C. Chambrier, A. Aouifi, C. Bon, F. Saudin, B. Paturel, P. Bouletreau, *J. Clin. Anesth.* 11, 646 (1999).

[16] E. S. Walsh, C. Traynor, J. L. Paterson, G. M. Hall, *Br. J. Anesth.* 55, 135 (1983).

[17] F. E. Sieber, D.S. Smith, R.J. Traystman, H. Wollman, 67, 72 (1987)

[18] C. Weissman, A*nesthesiology*, 73, 308 (1990).

[19] Zerr KJ, Furnary AP, Grunkemeier GL, Bookin S, Kanhere V, Starr A. Glucose control lowers the risk of wound infection in diabetics after open heart operations. *Ann. Thorac. Surg.* 1997;63:356-61.

[20] Ouattara, P. Lecomte, Y. Le Manach, M. Landi, S. Jacqueminet, I. Platonov, N. Bonnet, B. Riou, P. Coriat, *Anesthesiology,* 103, 687 (2005).

[21] D. L. Rothman, I. Magnusson, L.D. Katz, R.G. Shulman, G.I. Shulman, *Science,* 254, 573 (1991).

[22] K. M. Botham, Oxidation of fatty acids: Ketogenesis, 28th Edition Harper's illustrated biochemistry, Lange Medical Book, New York (2009).

[23] NICE SUGAR study investigators, N. Engl. J. Med. 360, 1283 (2009)

[24] T. Yokoyama, K. Suwa, F. Yamasaki, R Yokoyama, K. Yamashita, E. Sellden, Asia. *Pac. J. Clin. Nutr.* 17, 525 (2008).

[25] K. Yamasaki, Y. Inagaki, S. Mochida, K. Funaki, Takahashi, S. Sakamoto, *J. Anesth.* 24, 426 (2010).

[26] M. Mikura, I. Yamaoka, M. Doi, Y. Kawano, M. Nakayama, R. Nakao, K. Hirasaka, Y. Okumura, T .Nikawa, Anesthesiology, 110, 81 (2009)

[27] L.U. Monzillo, O. Hamdy, *Nutr. Rev.* 61, 397 (2003).

[28] Y. Tamura, Y. Tanaka, F. Sato, J.B. Choi, H. Watada, M. Niwa, J. Kinoshita, A. Ooka, N. Kumashiro, Y. Igarashi, S. Kyogoku, T. Maehara, M. Kawasumi, T. Hirose, R. Kawamori, *J. Clin. Endocrinol. Metab.* 90, 3191 (2005).

[29] F. Sato, Y. Tamura, H. Watada, N. Kumashiro, Y. Igarashi, H. Uchino, T. Maehara, S. Kyogoku, S. Sunayama, H. Sato, T. Hirose, Y. Tanaka, R. Kawamori, *J. Clin. Endocrinol. Metab.* 92, 3326 (2007).

[30] K. Nishida, S. Shimoda, K. Ichinose, E. Araki, M. Shichiri, *World J. Gastroenterol.* 15, 4105 (2009).

[31] K. Yamashita, T Okabayashi, T Yokoyama, T Yatabe, H Maeda, M Manabe, K Hanazaki, *Acta. Anaesthesiol. Scand.* 53, 66 (2009).

[32] K Yamashita, T. Okabayashi, T. Yokoyama, T. Yatabe, H. Maeda, M. Manabe, K. Hanazaki, *Anesth. Analg.* 106, 160 (2008).

[33] H. Fujino, S. Itoda, S. Sako, K. Matsuo, E. Sakamoto, T. Yokoyama, Masui. 62, 140 (2013).

[34] B. Baban, A. Thorell, J. Nygren, A. Bratt, O. Ljungqvist, *Clin. Nutr.* 34, 123 (2015).

[35] Y. Tsukamoto, Y. Kinoshita, H. Kitagawa, M. Munekage, E. Munekage, Y. Takezaki, T. Yatabe, K. Yamashita, R. Yamazaki, T. Okabayashi, M. Tarumi, M. Kobayashi, S. Mishina, K. Hanazaki, *Artif. Organs.* 37, E67 (2013).

[36] T. Yatabe, R. Yamazaki, H. Kitagawa, T. Okabayashi, K. Yamashita, K. Hanazaki, M. Yokoyama, *Crit. Care. Med.* 39, 575 (2011).

[37] T. Okabayashi, I. Nishimori, K. Yamashita, T. Sugimoto, H. Maeda, T. Yatabe, T. Kohsaki, M. Kobayashi, K. Hanazaki, *Arch. Surg.* 144, 933 (2009).

[38] H. Maeda, T. Okabayashi, T. Yatabe, K. Yamashita, K. Hanazaki, World *J. Gastroenterol.* 15, 4111 (2009).

[39] M. Emoto, Y. Nishizawa, K. Maekawa, T. Kawagishi, K. Kogawa, Y. Hiura, K. Mori, S. Tanaka, E. Ishimura, M. Inaba, Y. Okuno, H. Morii, *Metabolism.* 46, 1013 (1997).

[40] Thorell, J. Nygren, O. Ljungqvist, *Curr. Opin. Clin. Nutr. Metab. Care.* 2, 69 (1999).

[41] O. Ljungqvist, A. Thorell, M. Gutniak, T. Häggmark, S. Efendic, *J. Am. Coll. Surg.* 178, 329 (1994).

[42] M. Soop, J. Nygren, A. Thorell, L. Weidenhielm, M. Lundberg, F. Hammarqvist, O. Ljungqvist, *Clin. Nutr.* 23, 733 (2004).

[43] T. Tamura, T. Yatabe, H. Kitagawa, K. Yamashita, K. Hanazaki, M. Yokoyama, Asia. *Pac. J. Clin. Nutr.* 22, 48 (2013).

[44] T. Yatabe, T. Tamura, H. Kitagawa, T. Namikawa, K. Yamashita, K. Hanazaki, M. Yokoyama, *J. Artif. Organs.* 16, 483 (2013).

[45] H. Fujino, S. Itoda, K. Esaki, M. Tsukamoto, S. Sako, K. Matsuo, E. Sakamoto, K. Suwa, T. Yokoyama, Asia. *Pac. J. Clin. Nutr.* 23, 400 (2014).

[46] A. M. Roza, H.M. Shizgal, *Am. J. Clin. Nutr.* 40, 168 (1984).

[47] T. Yatabe, H. Kitagawa, K. Yamashita, K. Hanazaki, M. Yokoyama, Asia. *Pac. J. Clin. Nutr.* 23, 555 (2014).

[48] J. L. Gamble, the Harvey Lectures SERIES XLIII 1946-7, pp 247-273.

[49] L. Rubinson, G. B. Diette, X. Song, R. G. Brower, J. A. Krishnan, *Crit. Care. Med.* 32, 350 (2004).

[50] J. F. Patiño, S.E. de Pimiento, A. Vergara, P. Savino, M. Rodríguez, J. Escallón, *World J. Surg.* 23, 553 (1999).

[51] D. Mesotten, J. V. Swinnen, F. Vanderhoydonc, P. J. Wouters, G. Van den Berghe, *J. Clin. Endocrinol. Metab.* 89, 219 (2004).

[52] S. Dissanaike, M. Shelton, K. Warner, G. E. O'Keefe, *Crit. Care.* 11, R114 (2007).

[53] M. J. Sena, G.H. Utter, J. Cuschieri, R. V. Maier, R. G. Tompkins, B. G. Harbrecht, E. E. Moore, G. E. O'Keefe, *J. Am. Coll. Surg.* 207, 459 (2008).

[54] M. Svanfeldt, A. Thorell, J. Hausel, M. Soop, J. Nygren, O. Ljungqvist, *Clin. Nutr.* 24, 815 (2005).

[55] J. A. Calbet. D.A. MacLean, *J. Physiol.* 498, 553 (1997).

[56] D. L. Costill, B. Saltin, *J. Appl. Physiol.* 37, 679 (1974).

[57] G. E. Vist, R.J. Maughan, *Med. Sci. Sports Exerc.* 26, 1269 (1994)

[58] B. Brandstrup, P.E. Svendsen, M. Rasmussen, B. Belhage, S.Å. Rodt, B. Hansen, D.R. Møller, L.B. Lundbech, N. Andersen, V. Berg, N. Thomassen, S.T. Andersen, L. Simonsen, *Br. J. Anaesth.* 109, 191 (2012).

[59] P. Singer, M.M. Berger, G. Van den Berghe, G. Biolo, P. Calder, A. Forbes, R. Griffiths, G. Kreyman, X. Leverve, C. Pichard, ESPEN, *Clin. Nutr.* 28, 387 (2009).

[60] T. Schricker, M. Galeone, L. Wykes, F. Carli, *Acta. Anaesthesiol. Scand.* 48, 169 (2004).

[61] K. Watanabe, K. Kashiwagi, T. Kamiyama, M. Yamamoto, M. Fukunaga, E. Inada, Y. Kamiyama, *J. Anesth.* 28, 334 (2014).

[62] J. S. Krinsley, M. Egi, A. Kiss, A. N. Devendra, P. Schuetz, P. M. Maurer, M. J. Schultz, R. T. van Hooijdonk, M. Kiyoshi, I. M. Mackenzie, D. Annane, P. Stow, S.A. Nasraway, S. Holewinski, U. Holzinger, J. C. Preiser, J. L. Vincent, R. Bellomo, *Crit. Care.* 17, R37 (2013).

In: Impaired Glucose Tolerance ...   ISBN: 978-1-63483-085-0
Editor: Sandra Wagner   © 2015 Nova Science Publishers, Inc.

Chapter 4

Impaired Glucose Tolerance in Cystic Fibrosis

Peter G. Middleton[*,1], MBBS (Hons), BSc(Med), PhD, FRACP, FThorSoc,
Odette J. Erskine[2], MBBS (Hons), FRACP
and D. Jane Holmes-Walker[3], MBBS (Hons), PhD, FRACP

[1]Centre Director, [2] Respiratory & Sleep Physician,
[3]Endocrinologist, Adult CF Service, Westmead Hospital, Sydney, Australia

ABSTRACT

One of the major complications of Cystic Fibrosis (CF) is CF-related diabetes (CFRD) which increases in incidence with age, from 1-2% below the age of 10 years, to 25% in early adult life and over 50% in those above the age of 40 years. [1-3].

The diagnosis of CFRD is made clinically or through the Oral Glucose Tolerance Test (OGTT) which measures elevation of the fasting or 2 hour blood glucose levels. The diagnosis of Impaired Glucose

[*] Editorial correspondence: Peter G Middleton, Clinical Associate Professor, Ludwig Engel Centre for Respiratory Research, Westmead Millennium Institute, University of Sydney at Westmead, Westmead, NSW 2145, Australia, Ph: (+61 2) 9845 6797 Fax: (+61 2) 9845 7286, Email: peter.middleton@sydney.edu.au.

Tolerance (IGT) is made in those subjects with values between the normal and diabetic ranges. Outside of these definitions, abnormalities of the one hour glucose value of the OGTT may also be present. In this review, the significance of IGT in the management of CF will be reviewed and areas requiring further research to manage IGT in CF will be highlighted.

Keywords: impaired glucose tolerance, cystic fibrosis, diabetes

INTRODUCTION

Cystic Fibrosis (CF) is the most common lethal inherited disorder in Caucasians, affecting 1 in 2,500 - 2,800 live births[4]. CF results from mutations in the cystic fibrosis transmembrane conductance regulator gene (CFTR) which functions as a cyclic AMP-regulated chloride channel and as a regulator of other channels including the epithelial sodium channel (ENaC). The typical CF syndrome includes chronic suppurative lung disease, likely related to the decreased chloride secretion and increased sodium absorption characteristically found in the airways. CF also induces exocrine pancreatic insufficiency in most patients through pancreatic duct occlusion, which requires long term pancreatic enzyme supplementation, together with a high calorie diet, to maintain body weight.

One of the major complications of CF is CF-Related Diabetes (CFRD), the incidence of which increases with age, from 1-2% below the age of 10 years to more than 50% over the age of 40 years[1, 5]. As CFRD is associated with deteriorating lung function, increasing pulmonary infections, worsening nutritional status and ultimately increased mortality, it is now recommended that all CF patients should have an annual oral glucose tolerance test (OGTT) from the age of 10 years to screen for CFRD [6].

CFRD shares features of both Type I and Type II diabetes. The primary abnormality is progressive insulin deficiency, with multiple studies demonstrating impaired first phase insulin secretion [7, 8]. Interestingly, even in CF subjects with normal glucose tolerance, first phase insulin secretion may be delayed [9]. With age, the insulin secretory response progressively declines. Insulin sensitivity is variable among individuals with CF, with different studies demonstrating normal, increased or decreased insulin sensitivity, depending on glucose tolerance status [10, 11]. In addition to reduced beta cell mass and insulinopenia, increased gluconeogenesis with reduced suppression by insulin has been demonstrated in CF individuals [12]. Peripheral insulin resistance may be worsened by increased stress hormones such as catecholamines, cortisol and other inflammatory cytokines present during respiratory exacerbations, together with the effect of exogenous glucocorticoid therapy to treat the lung disease. Peripheral resistance may also be related to abnormal translocation of glucose transporter type 4 (GLUT-4) [13].

DIAGNOSIS OF CFRD – OGTT

While CFRD can be diagnosed based on an elevated fasting blood glucose level of ≥ 7.0mmol, this is usually a late event in the evolution of CFRD. Generally, the diagnosis of CFRD is made based on an abnormal OGTT on screening. The OGTT involves an overnight fast followed by ingestion of a standard glucose drink (1.75g/kg bodyweight, maximum 75g) with measurement of blood glucose at 0 and 120 minutes. The diagnosis of CFRD is established if the fasting glucose value is >7.0 mmol/L and/or the 2 hour value is >11.0mmol/L [6, 14]. If the 2 hour value is between 7.8 and 11.0 mmol/L this is defined as Impaired Glucose Tolerance (IGT). While it is accepted that CFRD is associated with deterioration in lung function [15, 16], the question remains at what level does elevation of blood glucose impact lung function. One study has found that CF subjects with IGT had worse pulmonary function as measured by spirometry compared with those who exhibited normal glucose tolerance [17]. Although poor glycaemic control in established CFRD is associated with more frequent exacerbations of CF lung disease, which improve following insulin [18], the role of insulin in IGT is still unclear.

Over the last 10 years, CFRD is increasingly being recognised as a cause of microvascular complications [19]. This likely reflects both an increased diagnosis of CFRD and longer overall survival following the diagnosis of CFRD. Whilst renal disease is seen in CFRD, at present the prevalence of macrovascular disease is less than other diabetic populations, likely reflecting interactions with other vascular risk factors such as smoking, hypercholesterolemia etc.

New Research

Currently, the literature has not adequately addressed the optimal time to commence insulin in patients with CFRD, nor whether there is any benefit prescribing insulin therapy for IGT. Whilst it is agreed that insulin should be given for CFRD irrespective of fasting hyperglycemia [6, 20], the situation for CF patients with IGT is less clear. A small case series of 4 patients with IGT [21], did show some apparent benefit, but in the Moran et al. study [20], the group of patients with IGT (n=20) did not show any benefit with insulin. Thus, at present, the benefit versus risk ratio for insulin therapy in those with IGT is not clear.

The ramifications of a diagnosis of CFRD for those CF patients with no clinical symptoms, stable lung function and an isolated elevation of the 2 hour blood glucose is unclear and needs to be balanced with the risks of diagnosis and therapy. Insulin therapy adds to the therapeutic burden in CF so evidence of clinical benefit needs to be shown. Studies are required to examine the effect of insulin in CF subjects with asymptomatic IGT.

The Indeterminate GTT

Recently, the question has been raised whether measuring blood glucose values fasting and 2 hour post glucose load are sufficient for evaluation of CFRD. A number of groups have demonstrated marked elevations of BGL at 30 to 60 minutes following glucose load, consistent with loss of first phase insulin secretion, but normal blood glucose values at 120 minutes, hence by current definition "normal" glucose tolerance. We and others have been examining the outcome of this so called "indeterminate" glucose tolerance to assess whether loss of first phase insulin secretion and consequent abnormalities early in the OGTT are associated with any measurable change in respiratory or nutrition outcomes in CF (Erskine *et al* in preparation). Recently Brodsky *et al* performed a cross-sectional study comparing clinical variables in groups of children with transient elevations of the 1 hour blood glucose value during OGTT testing [22]. The group with a 1 hour value of >11.1 mmol (200 mg/dL) had a worse FEV_1 compared with those who had lower one hour values. However, the OGTT was only measured on a single day, and not repeated. As glucose tolerance acutely worsens during a pulmonary exacerbation [23], the question remains whether the worse pulmonary function was due to the presence of impaired glucose tolerance or whether the impaired glucose tolerance and worse FEV$_1$ simply reflected a mild pulmonary exacerbation. This also raises the problem of timing of the OGTT in subjects who have recurrent respiratory exacerbations, as acute respiratory exacerbations and other illness at the time of testing may worsen the OGTT results.

Thus it remains unclear whether indeterminate glucose tolerance has an impact on respiratory function in both the short and long term.

FURTHER RESEARCH

Several studies have shown that IGT does not necessarily proceed to CFRD as a continuum, as is generally seen in the non-CF population. While early studies [24] suggested that over a 14 year period of follow-up of the same individuals, glucose tolerance deteriorated over time, others [25] have since shown that glucose intolerance is not always progressive with serial yearly OGTT. The OGTT can return to normal glucose tolerance from IGT without treatment. The presence of intercurrent infection, poor nutrition and / or lack of muscle bulk are associated with impairments of glucose tolerance, yet with attention to treatment of infection, improved nutrition and muscle bulk, the OGTT may return towards the normal range on repeat testing.

In the recent past, many CF patients were advised to use sugar-containing beverages to maintain caloric intake and thus maintain body mass index. Whether the use of these high GI foods in childhood has any impact on progression to CFRD through contributions to beta cell stress and attrition is not known. Additional research is required into the impact of dietary manipulation on the risk of developing CFRD.

Finally, if less severe elevations of blood glucose adversely affect respiratory outcomes, then CFRD may require different OGTT criteria for diagnosis. Should the cut-points between the normal range, impaired glucose tolerance and diabetes for the 2 hour level of the OGTT be 7.8 and 11.0, or should the upper limit of the normal range for the 2 hour value be at a lower value? This would be analogous to gestational diabetes, where lower glucose cut off values are used during pregnancy to minimise adverse outcomes on the foetus. New technology such as continuous glucose monitoring is altering the way we investigate and manage glucose tolerance in both non-CF and CF related diabetes. The possibility of establishing criteria for diagnosis of CFRD from continuous glucose monitoring requires further research.

In summary, the recent data suggests that progression to CFRD may be modifiable, with progression potentially prevented by addressing pro-diabetogenic factors such as pulmonary exacerbations, use of steroid therapy and loss of muscle mass, and diabetes specific measures such as dietary modification. The exact timing of insulin therapy needs more evidence to guide the CF endocrinologist and CF respiratory physician.

CONCLUSION

In the CF population, it is reasonably well established that CF-related diabetes results in adverse outcomes, with both pulmonary and nutritional decline contributing to increased morbidity and mortality. However, the presence of impaired glucose tolerance needs to be studied further to determine its impact on nutritional and pulmonary outcomes. The question remains whether there is a threshold of glucose abnormality at which CF management is impacted or if there is a linear relationship between the 2 hour glucose and pulmonary outcomes analogous to the impact of the 2 hour glucose on the foetus [26].

If IGT is associated with adverse outcomes then randomised trials with insulin will need to be performed in large numbers of CF subjects to assess benefit. Only then can recommendations be made for the management of IGT and indeterminate glucose tolerance, to ensure we do not inappropriately increase the burden of therapy in our CF population.

REFERENCES

[1]   Moran A, Hardin D, Rodman D, et al. Diagnosis, screening and management of cystic fibrosis related diabetes mellitus: a consensus conference report. *Diab. Res. Clin. Pract.* 1999: 45: 61-73.

[2]   Rana M, Munns CF, Selvadurai HC, et al. Increased detection of cystic-fibrosis-related diabetes in Australia. *Arch. Dis. Child* 2011: 96(9): 823-826.

[3]   Moran A, Becker D, Casella SJ, et al. Epidemiology, pathophysiology, and prognostic implications of cystic fibrosis-related diabetes: a technical review. *Diabetes Care* 2010: 33(12): 2677-2683.

[4]   Bell SC, Bye PT, Cooper PJ, et al. Cystic fibrosis in Australia, 2009: results from a data registry. *Med. J. Aust.* 2011: 195(7): 396-400.

[5]   Moran A, Dunitz J, Nathan B, et al. Cystic fibrosis-related diabetes: current trends in prevalence, incidence, and mortality. *Diabetes Care* 2009: 32: 1626-1631.

[6]   Moran A, Brunzell C, Cohen RC, et al. Clinical care guidelines for cystic fibrosis-related diabetes: a position statement of the American Diabetes Association and a clinical practice guideline of the Cystic Fibrosis Foundation, endorsed by the Pediatric Endocrine Society. *Diabetes Care* 2010: 33: 2697-2708.

[7]   Handwerger S, Roth J, Gorden P, et al. Glucose intolerance in cystic fibrosis. *N. Engl. J. Med.* 1969: 281: 451-461.

[8]   Milner AD. Blood glucose and serum insulin levels in children with cystic fibrosis. *Arch. Dis. Child* 1969: 44: 351-355.

[9]   Moran A, Diem P, Klein DJ, Levitt MD, Robertson RP. Pancreatic endocrine function in cystic fibrosis. *J. Pediatr.* 1991: 118: 715-723.

[10]   Moran A, Pyzdrowski KL, Weinreb J, et al. Insulin sensitivity in cystic fibrosis. *Diabetes* 1994: 43: 1020-1026.

[11]   Hardin DS, LeBlanc A, Lukenbough S, Seilheimer DK. Insulin resistance is associated with decreased clinical status in cystic fibrosis. *J. Pediatr.* 1997: 130: 948-956.

[12]   Hardin DS, Ahn C, Rice J, Rice M, Rosenblatt R. Elevated gluconeogenesis and lack of suppression by insulin contribute to cystic fibrosis-related diabetes. *J. Investig. Med.* 2008: 56: 567-573.

[13]   Hardin DS, Leblanc A, Marshall G, Seilheimer DK. Mechanisms of insulin resistance in cystic fibrosis. *Am. J. Physiol. Endocrinol. Metab.* 2001: 281: E1022-1028.

[14]   Middleton PG, Wagenaar M, Matson AG, et al. Australian standards of care for cystic fibrosis-related diabetes. *Respirol* 2014: 19(2): 185-192.

[15]   Finkelstein SM, Wielinski CL, Elliott GR, et al. Diabetes mellitus associated with cystic fibrosis. *J. Pediatr.* 1988: 112: 373-377.

[16]   Koch C, Cuppens H, Rainisio M, et al. European Epidemiologic Registry of Cystic Fibrosis (ERCF): comparison of major disease manifestations between patients with different classes of mutations. *Pediatr. Pulmonol.* 2001: 31: 1-12.

[17]   Milla CE, Warwick WJ, Moran A. Trends in pulmonary function in patients with cystic fibrosis correlate with the degree of glucose intolerance at baseline. *Am. J. Respir. Crit. Care Med.* 2000: 162: 891-895.

[18]   Lanng S, Thorsteinsson B, Nerup J, Koch C. Diabetes mellitus in cystic fibrosis: effect of insulin therapy on lung function and infections. *Acta Paediatrica* 1994: 83: 849-853.

[19]   van den Berg JMW, Morton AM, Kok SW, et al. Microvascular complications in patients with cystic fibrosis-related diabetes (CFRD). *J. Cyst. Fibros.* 2008: 7(6): 515-519.

[20]   Moran A, Pekow P, Grover P, et al. Insulin therapy to improve BMI in cystic fibrosis-related diabetes without fasting hyperglycemia. *Diabetes Care* 2009: 32: 1783-1788.

[21]   Dobson L, Hattersley AT, Tiley S, et al. Clinical improvement in cystic fibrosis with early insulin treatment. *Arch. Dis. Child* 2002: 87(5): 430-431.

[22]   Brodsky J, Dougherty S, Makani R, Rubenstein RC, Kelly A. Elevation of 1-hour plasma glucose during oral glucose tolerance testing is associated with worse pulmonary function in cystic fibrosis. *Diabetes Care* 2011: 34(2): 292-295.

[23]   Sc NN, Shoseyov D, Kerem E, Zangen DH. Patients with cystic fibrosis and normoglycemia exhibit diabetic glucose tolerance during pulmonary exacerbation. *J. Cyst. Fibros.* 2010: 9: 199-204.

[24]   Lombardo F, De Luca F, Rosano M, et al. Natural history of glucose tolerance, beta-cell function and peripheral insulin sensitivity in cystic fibrosis patients with fasting euglycemia. *Eur. J. Endocrinol.* 2003: 149: 53-59.

[25]   Sterescu AE, Rhodes B, Jackson R, et al. Natural history of glucose intolerance in patients with cystic fibrosis: ten-year prospective observation program. *J. Pediatr.* 2010: 156(4): 613-617.

[26]   Landon MB, Spong CY, Thom E, et al. A multicenter, randomized trial of treatment for mild gestational diabetes. *N. Engl. J. Med.* 2009: 361: 1339-1348.

Index

F

G

H